Notes from the Waiting Room

Managing a Loved One's End-of-Life Hospitalization

INCLUDES:
Choosing
End-of-Life Care
Without
Hospitalization

BART WINDRUM

www.NotesFromTheWaitingRoom.com
www.WaitingRoomBook.com
www.AxiomAction.com

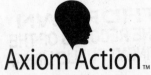

Axiom Action™

Discounted bulk purchases are available. Contact Axiom Action, LLC, at 1-888-5-WAITING or Bulk@AxiomAction.com.

Other books by Bart Windrum:
How to Efficiently Settle the Family Estate

Publisher's Cataloging-In-Publication Data

Notes from the waiting room: managing a loved one's end-of-life hospitalization / Bart Windrum.
xvi, 336p. 23cm.
Includes bibliographical references and index.
ISBN-13 978-0-9801090-0-9
ISBN-10 0-9801090-0-0
1. Terminal Care 2. Hospital Care 3. Death
4. Hospitals—Moral and Ethical Aspects I. Title II. Author
R726.8.W56 2008   362.175—dc22
Library of Congress Control Number: 2007942494

Printed in Canada on 100% post-consumer recycled paper.

Book Design	Axiom Action, LLC
Typefaces	ITC Stone Serif and Stone Sans, ITC New Baskerville, Sunflower, SBC Distressed Typewriter
Cover Design	George Foster

Notes
from the
Waiting
Room

Managing a Loved One's End-of-Life Hospitalization

INCLUDES:
Choosing
End-of-Life Care
Without
Hospitalization

For my mother Ruth—
We had a gracious plenty

For my father Mort—
His spirit lifted ours

For you—
When assuming the role of personal representative
on behalf of your hospitalized or dying loved one,
I wish you the grace my mother manifested at her finest,
the uplift my father produced in all
who encountered him during his last decades,
the empowerment to enter this crucible with resolve,
and the wherewithal to emerge from the crucible
with your spirit strengthened.

CONTENTS

Thoughts for Those in Acute Need or Crisis......................... xii

New Terms for a Clear Conversation 19

Preface | The Genesis of *Notes from the Waiting Room*................... 29

The Experiences Behind This Book   29
Interviewees   32
The Theses and Their Validation   36
Not About Blame   37
Dissatisfaction Clarified   38
Disclaimers   39
For the Record: A Litany of Problems   40

Introduction.. 45

An Antidote to Profoundly Serious Problems   45
Understanding "The System"   46
Assumptions   47
Range, Focus, and Exclusions   48
A Zillion Variables   51
Defining Families   51
Exposing the Unexposed   52
Several Unexpectedly Big Topics   52
Emotional Understanding and the Urgency to Act   53

Section 1 | EFFECTIVELY REPRESENT YOUR LOVED ONE................. 55

1 | Be an Effective Personal Representative 57

For Those In Acute Need or Crisis   60
What is a Personal Representative?   62
Why is a Personal Representative Needed in Hospitals Today?   63
What Makes a Personal Representative Effective?   63
Why is Effective Personal Representation Important? 72
How to Get Comfortable in the Role of Question-Asker 74
Personal Representative Recap: What You Can Do   76

2 | Making Effective Declarations:
The Essential Power Documents **77**

For Those In Acute Need or Crisis   79
The Only Way to Make Effective and Binding Declarations   81
The Medical Durable Power of Attorney Document   84
The HIPAA Authorization and Release Document   85
The Living Will (Advance Directive) Document   86
The Do Not Resuscitate (DNR) Form   88
The Financial Durable Power of Attorney Document   89
Other Legal Documents: Wills and Trusts   90
What Makes Power Documents Effective?   90
The Size of the Law Firm and Power Documents   93
Power Documents Recap: What You Can Do   94

Section 2 | EFFECTIVELY MANAGE HOSPITALIZATION **95**

3 | Differing Sensibilities:
Care and Communication in Hospitals **99**

For Those In Acute Need or Crisis   101
The Significance of Communication and the Shock of its Absence   103
Redefining Hospitals   104
How Hospitals Compare   107
Why We Expect Care From Hospitals   108
Redefining the Patient   113
What We Really Need to Know from Hospitals   115
Hospital Care and Communication Recap: What You Can Do   116

4 | Family Involvement in Hospital Care **117**

For Those In Acute Need or Crisis   119
Why Hospitals are the Way They Are   121
Several Well-known Hospitalization Risks   125
The Need to Oversee Your Loved One's Treatment   126
"Family Care" Means Your Family Provides the Care   126
The Family-Friendly Hospital Environment   127
Where Treatment Discussions and Conferences Take Place   128
Discontinuity of Care and Discontinuity of Communication   129
Who Not to Complain To and What to Know if You Do   131
Who Pays How Much for What?   134
Family Involvement in Hospital Care Recap: What You Can Do   136

5 | Forecasting and Ethical Support: What You Need to Know, When You Need to Know It, and How to Get It **137**

For Those In Acute Need or Crisis   139

The Significance of Forecasting and the Shock of its Absence   141

Ethical Support Services to Assist with Forecasting   149

Forecasting and Ethical Support Summary   157

Forecasting and Ethical Support Recap: What You Can Do   158

6 | Who's Where, When, Why, for How Long, and Other Turns through the Hospital Maze **159**

For Those In Acute Need or Crisis   162

Hospital Time   164

Who Is That Administering to Your Loved One?   167

Firing Nurses, Doctors, and Hospitals   170

Hospitalization Experienced as a Crucible   175

Who's Where, When, Why, for How Long, and Other Turns
    Through the Hospital Maze Recap: What You Can Do   177

7 | The Complete Do-Not-Resuscitate Conversation **179**

For Those In Acute Need or Crisis   183

The Complete Do-Not-Resuscitate Conversation   185

Resuscitation and its Relationship with Treatment Goals   187

Practicalities and Legalities of Resuscitation   189

The Ethical Gray Zones Around Resuscitation   196

Future Resuscitation Choices   209

Resuscitation Conclusion and Recommendations   210

Resuscitation Recap: What You Can Do   212

Section 3 | THE IMPERATIVE TO CHANGE END OF LIFE **215**

8 | Death Looks Like This **219**

For Those In Acute Need or Crisis   220

Why an Accurate Depiction of Death Matters   222

My Father's Remains   223

Spirituality and Corpses   225

What Might You Encounter?   226

The Psyche Must be Fed   227

Signals that Death May Be Near   231

Handling the Body   236

Funeral Arrangements   238

Changing Our Experience of Death   239

Death Looks Like This Recap: What You Can Do   239

9 | The Option to Die in PEACE:
Patient Ethical Alternative Care Elective **241**

For Those In Acute Need or Crisis   243
Existing End-of-Life Options   248
The Surprising Nature of Hospital Death   255
Taking Control of Our Deaths: The Option to Die in PEACE   258
Overcoming the Obstacles to PEACE   260
Dying at Home, in Home-Like Communities, or Hospice   268
Reframing Heroic Action   269
It's Up to Us: the Imperative for PEACE is Personal   273
The Option to Die in PEACE Recap: What You Can Do   277

Section 4 | TOWARD HEAVENLY DAYS.......................... **279**

10 | Epilogue and Proposals for Medical System Reform........... **281**

Physician Training and Licensure Reform   284
Hospital Administrative Reform   285
Patient-Family Resources Reform   285
Patient-Family Treatment Reform   286
Patient-Family Autonomy Reform   290

11 | Thoughts for Medical Providers........................... **291**

Afterword | The Moving Medical Target **295**

Acknowledgments **299**

Recommended Reading **303**

The Best of the Best   303
The Rest of the Best   306

Endnotes... **309**

Index **319**

Notes
from the
Waiting
Room

THOUGHTS FOR THOSE IN ACUTE NEED OR CRISIS

MAYBE YOU'RE FREAKED OUT. Your loved one is hospitalized. Maybe it's a surprise, a shock. Maybe s/he's in critical condition in an intensive care unit (ICU). Maybe terminal. Maybe there's a decision you have to make -- perhaps a life-and-death decision. How prepared are you to make it?

You and your family assemble at the hospital -- a foreboding environment. A teeming, technical, yet bland place where time moves strangely and what lies ahead is not explained. You're left alone with your languishing loved one, your uncertainties, doubts, and fears.

To ensure that your family's best interests are served, you must proactively unearth all kinds of information by asking endless questions, up front, of virtually every person who interacts with you in a professional capacity. To ensure that your loved one doesn't languish, you must have that information before each next choice point -- some moment that practically begs for a decision. How do you get it? How do you know what to ask for? How do you anticipate when the next choice point may occur?

If this loved one is your last living parent, and if s/he dies, you may have the double task of closing the parental home and beginning to settle the family estate. A task that, depending upon circumstances, may not be able to wait another day if you're half a continent from your own life and home. The need to begin this work may arise even as your loved one lies dying.

THIS BOOK OFFERS A COMPILATION OF GUIDANCE YOU WON'T FIND ELSEWHERE. My experience during and after two terminal hospitalizations taught me that healthcare establishments neither talk about nor offer the information you most need to know -- especially what you need to know to help you in your hours and days of need, whether your loved one is terminal or hospitalized for less severe conditions. To the limited extent that institutions talk about matters vital to you, their communication is not offered in advance; it usually coincides with some disconcerting or agonizing choice point.

If you are your loved one's designated personal representative (known also as proxy, agent, surrogate, or Medical Power of Attorney) and your family's values are like mine, communing with your loved one, receiving direction from your loved one, and avoiding detrimental emotional shocks are among your family's most vital interests.

You may need help in making a life-and-death decision. But if you're not sure what death's onset looks like, you won't know that a life-and-death decision may be looming.

Unless you happen across an "angel"[1] in the hospital halls or during telephone calls, you may be at the mercy of people who, for various reasons, do not offer ample guidance, or any guidance, or don't even do their job well. Perhaps they do their job well but their job definition or professional orientation is limited in scope and doesn't reach as far as providing the kind of care families expect for their loved ones -- the kind of care we provide for one another.

During two hospitalizations fifteen months apart and totaling almost six weeks, my family received virtually zero advance notice of things to come, let alone any guidance. Without notification of what was likely or possible to happen, we experienced repeated, deep, destabilizing -- and unnecessary -- shocks. Our equilibrium suffered, and important opportunities were foreclosed, vanishing opportunities to commune with and receive treatment direction from our loved ones. Without guidance, our best interests were not served by providers or by institutional staff and representatives. Rather, we had to discover for ourselves how to have our best interests served, moment by moment, time and again -- during the most urgent, stressful, and vulnerable of times of our lives.

Thus, this book. WITHIN A FEW HOURS' READING, YOU'LL LEARN WHAT IT TOOK US MONTHS TO LEARN AND PIECE TOGETHER from disparate sources (years, actually, if we include my subsequent research and contemplation). Through these pages, you and I will converse in the peace and quiet of your own reading environment. Unlike my family, YOU WON'T HAVE TO LEARN SOLELY ON THE SPUR OF THE MOMENT, when unexpected choices are conveyed with no prior notice. As if they would not rock your world. As if the choices before you weren't emotional bombs. As if the casual notification of the need to choose didn't add additional shock to the cataclysmic, intrinsic shock of a loved one down, possibly on their deathbed.

IF YOU ARE IN CRISIS, if right now is your spur-of-the-moment, I wish I could sit with you and help you personally. This book will have to be my stand-in. Although writing a book is primarily a mental exercise, I have tried to imbue this one with heart and soul; I hope that at times you can sense their presence and feel bolstered.

TO SAVE TIME, you may want to skip our italicized stories that begin each chapter. If you need infor-

mation you can act on right now and are inclined to consider my suggestions without substantiation, read each
chapter's "notes," summarizations that look like this
following each chapter's opening story. Then read sections that address your most pressing concerns.

Afterward, when you have the time, I suggest you read
our stories. The snapshots describe events that occurred
to my family and which could occur to yours. Our stories
are vital to a complete understanding of the narrative;
they will help you identify, understand, and overcome
needlessly stressful situations associated with serious
hospitalizations -- especially those that turn terminal.

Godspeed --

T HE NIGHT MY FATHER DIED, *her connecting flight was delayed. She was aboard a conveyance that takes untold millions of living human beings as close to the heavens as all but a very few will go during our earthly existence.*

My wife returned to earth, we surmise, at the very moment that Dad's newly-freed spirit may have been making a voyage in exactly the opposite direction (assuming, that is, that newly-freed spirits exist and have, or even need, a sense of direction).

Deborah's plane was scheduled to land in south Florida at 11:30 p.m. Due to a passenger emergency, it made an unscheduled stop en route. Our original plan had me picking her up at the airport and driving to Dad's nearby hospice room for their last communion. I had stayed at his bedside later than usual, but after learning of the delay, I piloted Dad's van through the seventeen-mile drive to his assisted living apartment, where I'd been living for the previous two weeks. There, I did another round of endless tasks associated with closing a home half a continent from my own—jockeying the phone, notes to myself, financial files, online research, legal queries, property dispositions, a canned dinner. I fell asleep on the floor; my dad's hospital-style bed had been returned to Medicare.

Almost immediately, the phone rang. The hospice nurse breathlessly told me that my dad's own breathing had unexpectedly changed to end stage. In her experience, his passing might occur at any moment, even though its imminence caught her by surprise. Well, that was my father, I reflected. He was a black-and-white type of guy who did not engage in subtleties, and his dying process mirrored that in this seemingly sudden turn toward the end.

I made the midnight drive back on empty boulevards, speeding a little but not as much as I would have liked. I didn't want to risk being pulled over and further delayed. The hospital parking lot, full to capacity during the daytime, was barren now as I slipped his van into the spot closest to the entrance.

Grimly, I hiked up several flights of stairs and strode through the labyrinthine hallways I'd come to learn as if they were my new neighborhood. In the soundless hospice wing, the solitary nurse approached and told me my father had died twenty minutes earlier.

She expected me to want her hug—or to want to hug her. Maybe she needed that hug, or to give it, and I regretted that I didn't have it in me. I didn't share that thought with her, although I wondered in that moment if she thought me deficient as she stiffened from my unavailability. In retrospect, I surmise that at her lonely post, a midnight guardian of those who die, she needed a respite from unavailability and stiffness, hallmarks of the remains of the newly departed.

I was not present at my mom's passing fifteen months prior, and by the time I'd flown in, her remains were ashes. I'd never seen or encountered human death. I'd never experienced the evidence death leaves behind. I'd only experienced the absences of living far away from family visited once or twice a year and old friends seen once or twice a decade.

Had circumstances been different, my wife and I would have been present when Dad died, to be with him as his spirit took its leave. Instead, nineteen days after taking himself into the hospital, twenty minutes after his passing, I entered my father's room alone.

New Terms for a Clear Conversation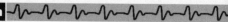

New Terms To Define Hospital Experiences

NOTES FROM THE WAITING ROOM DISSECTS EVENTS you may encounter during a loved one's hospitalization and death. If things are to go poorly, chances are this will occur during the last weeks and days of your loved one's life. Since approximately fifty percent of Americans die in hospitals,[2] *Notes from the Waiting Room* focuses on what happens in that setting.

During this conversation I introduce a variety of new terms. Familiarity with these terms is key to understanding what can occur when loved ones' lives end in hospitals and the nature of hospitalization as we experience it.

As far as I know only two of these terms are, at the time of this writing, in general use in the medical world: discontinuity of care and time-based trial.

While a list of definitions might seem like an unusual way to begin a book, this list actually summarizes much of what *Notes from the Waiting Room* has to offer. The group of terms as a whole provides a framework for an in-depth discussion of hospitalization in general, and end-of-life experience in particular, whether in the hospital or elsewhere.

In addition to clarifying things, the right terminology serves two other important purposes. First, naming an experience helps us make meaning of it. Once we begin making meaning of experiences, we can better assess what we've been through. We can begin to figure out how systems function. Second, naming an experience offers several important personal benefits. Our experience is validated; we're not crazy or wrong. We realize that we're not isolated; we're not alone, either in our experience or our understanding of it. Naming an experience serves to formalize and normalize it (i.e., to see something as common rather than as an exception). Once we understand that our experiences are normal, we can examine institutional and societal behavior from a place of confidence, rather than sheepishly feeling that something is wrong with us for having "gotten ourselves" into some problem situation.

Opting to use new terminology makes us proactive proponents, and components, of change within the system. For example, when providers and institutions start hearing us refer to ourselves as "patient-families" again and again, they can't help but begin to modify their viewpoint of their customer base. When we inject the term "forecasting" into our conversations in doctors' offices and at the bedside, a new level of consciousness and attentiveness is bound to arise over time. Ask and ye shall receive.

With this in mind, here's my list of new terms and concepts to use when discussing the continuum of experiences during hospitalization and end-of-life.

Redefining Hospitals

The dictionary defines hospitals as places providing medical or surgical care. The trouble is that hospitals and lay people define care differently. This mismatch results in turmoil and anxiety when people experience what hospitals and providers consider to be care. Thus, it's useful to explicitly define what hospitals offer. Aside from Emergency Department services and walk-in clinics, in the context of serious and/or extended hospitalizations, *hospitals provide bodily repair services under the direction of independent physician-scientists.*

Independent Physician-Scientist

With few exceptions, doctors and surgeons are self-employed (typically as part of a small business group); they are not employees of the several hospitals at which they practice. While responsible to their patients, they answer essentially to themselves, their business partners, and their colleagues.

Have no doubt that they are scientists. Their training is disciplined and arduous, and the best doctors innovate, developing disease-solving, life-extending products and techniques. These vital skills are different from those associated with healing.[3]

Some doctors may cringe upon hearing that they practice bodily repair, or even loathe the assertion. Those who take exception apparently mistake the phrase as a contention that they are simply technicians, a real slight in that techs rank much lower than physicians in the medical hierarchy. And for good reason: techs undergo a fraction of the training required of doctors. However, if physicians are able to set aside the devaluation they feel and think objectively, they may nod in agreement that this phrase fairly represents their outlook, function, and performance. It may not reflect the highest ideals espoused at the beginning of their medical training, but those ideals have in most cases been trained away in medical school, and drained away in the workplace due to the pressures of practicing medicine in an environment controlled by the insurance industry and large corporations.

Patient-Family

The patient-family is the unit (customer) deserving of caring attention during a loved one's hospitalization. Caring for the patient involves diagnoses, clinical treatment, and attentiveness to their well-being, plus caring for the family. Caring for the family involves a family-friendly environment and policies, ongoing forecasting (see below), and ethical assistance if desired.[4] Family care ought to be part of every hospitalization if only because of the central role families are now called upon to play there. Your comfort level with this term may grow; I find myself using the word "patient" alone under very narrow circumstances.

Treatment Group

The treatment group is comprised of the medical providers who attend to a hospitalized patient-family. "Treatment group" replaces the traditional phrase "care team." Since the notion of care has morphed into bodily repair, and treatment may not be as closely coordinated as the word "team" connotes, *treatment group* more accurately conveys the range of services available to patient-families in their felt experience.

Specialists often function on a level field without a clear go-to team lead. "Team" connotes a working process tightly coordinated under a clear chain of command. This goal goes unmet enough of the time to warrant a name for it within the medical establishment: discontinuity of care.

Note: treatment group ought not be confused with the formal business arrangement of a group practice, e.g., "Some Medical Office, LLC."

Discontinuity of Care

Discontinuity of care is the industry name given when gaps occur in the administration and oversight of patient treatment. I expand it to include gaps in communication with the family—whether those gaps are the result of provider or institutional failure. As we'll see, communication that does not occur, or occurs poorly, is a primary cause of negative results ranging from repetitive needless duress to medical error.

"Care" and "caregiver" are terms for which substitutes currently do not exist. Critics have suggested that we don't really have a health-care system but, rather, a disease-care system. This book challenges the notion that hospitals provide *any* care[5] during serious hospitalizations. I have tried to minimize the use of these words in this book, substituting *provider* for caregiver and *treatment* for care, whenever possible (which is, in general, but a fraction of the time; the word "care" is unalterably embedded throughout medical terminology).

Personal Representative

As a personal representative, you assume one or two legally empowered roles assigned by a loved one, on his or her behalf. Made effective by signed legal documents, the agent named in a Medical Power of Attorney advocates for and makes binding healthcare decisions; the agent named in a Property (or

Financial) Power of Attorney conducts financial and contractual affairs.

Various terms are used to refer to the person(s) representing a patient and the power given that person, so we ought to clarify to avoid confusion.

One point of confusion could arise in hospitals between *personal representative* and *patient liaison* (or *patient advocate*). Hospitals may employ people with the title of "patient liaison" or "patient advocate." While it's vital that you proactively advocate for your loved one's benefit (because their well-being—perhaps life—depends upon your advocacy), it's important that we differentiate the hospital-employed advocate from you, your loved one's personal representative.

To me, using the term *personal representative* to refer to a family member or close friend representing a loved one during hospitalization is clearly apt. The role is deeply *personal*, and you *represent* your loved one regarding vital matters. And although *patient representative* might suffice within the hospital, the term *personal representative* works in both the medical and financial context—each of which are relevant, especially at end of life, which can extend beyond hospitalization through estate settlement.[6]

In any case, whatever the terms used on the scene to describe your role while representing your loved one's wishes, the treatment group will know who you are and what your authority consists of.

A second confusion could arise in the financial realm, but only in select locales. In terms of medical and financial matters, the United States is 50 jurisdictions governed by 50 sets of laws (further subdivided into more than 3,000 county jurisdictions). In certain jurisdictions, "personal representative" means the person named as Financial Power of Attorney, who is legally empowered to execute the family estate, to buy and sell, obtain and distribute assets.

Forecasting

Forecasting is the provision of advance information or notice about possible events to come. This is a word used in medical ethics.[7] Don't expect doctors and nurses to know or use "forecasting" (although they will probably understand its meaning quickly when you use it). Doctors' prognoses, which forecast possible patient outcomes, are a subset of forecasting. My use of the term includes up-front information from hospitals, insurers, and financial institutions about how their systems work, what to expect as we engage with them, and what's in our best interest based on our particulars. The point of forecasting is to eliminate extrinsic shock.

Intrinsic Shock

Intrinsic shock is the shock that we experience due to something's essential nature. Intrinsic shock is inherent to the situation. Example: your loved one is hospitalized in intensive care. You are shocked to learn this. Upon arrival in the ICU, you are further shocked to see your loved one with all the medical paraphernalia attached—intravenous tubes connected to drips and various machines with multiple displays and readouts. The shock you feel is intrinsic, due to the fact of your loved one's condition, hospitalization, uncertainty, and risk.

Extrinsic Shock

Extrinsic shock is the shock that comes not as a natural result of a situation but in addition to it. We experience extrinsic shock due to something external to whatever has caused our intrinsic shock. Example: information about your loved one's condition that could have been shared with you is not. When that information is finally shared with you, it may be delivered casually, with no preliminaries, and in the context of an imminent procedure or important decision. Because of all of this, you feel shocked, perhaps emotionally pained. Your equilibrium (such as it is in these circumstances) is sent into a wobble. Procedures and decisions may be put on hold while you take one or more days to sort out the complexities in your own mind and heart, with your loved one and/or family members. Meanwhile your loved one languishes needlessly, because aspects related to his condition could have been forecast during the several days prior to the choice point, during which family deliberations (and communion) could have occurred.

Communion

Communion is defined by the dictionary as *the sharing or exchanging of intimate thoughts and feelings.* During critical hospitalizations, or those which could turn critical (i.e., any hospitalization), opportunities for communion with a loved one are precious. A lack of forecasting undermines patient-families who may not recognize that these opportunities could be or are diminishing. During end of life, these missed opportunities cannot be reclaimed. Communion includes opportunities to discuss and receive treatment direction from your loved one. If you fail to obtain this, you may well end up making a "pull-the-plug" decision yourself, as did my sister and I.

Time-based Trial

A time-based trial[8] is the explicit allowance of a specific medical treatment for a limited period of time that's been negotiated and agreed upon in advance by the parties involved. If the treatment is still being administered at the end of this period, doctors agree to cease it when directed by, and based on prior agreement with, the patient or personal representative. Example: a patient with a Do Not Resuscitate order undergoes minor surgery to correct some problem. There's a small chance of life-support being required post-op. Being on life-support is against the patient's Living Will and Do Not Resuscitate status, but will be tolerated by the patient-family on a time-based trial basis only for a previously agreed upon duration.

Power Documents

Power Documents are the set of legal documents that together form the framework for one's formal expression of medical and financial desires. These documents typically designate a person (or persons) to represent the person drafting them, with full legal authority, when one cannot represent oneself. The Power Documents are:

- Living Will (advance directive)
- HIPAA Authorization and Release (HIPAA is the acronym for the federal government's Health Insurance Portability and Accountability Act, responsible for several well-known reforms, including health insurance maintenance options for people losing or changing jobs, and for the myriad of health information privacy initiatives and policies).
- Medical Durable Power of Attorney

- Property (financial) Durable Power of Attorney
- Do Not Resuscitate (DNR) Form (and/or DNR order).[9]

After these documents have been correctly executed and are in effect (based on circumstances and how the documents are worded), and when they are presented to medical and financial officials, the named personal representative (usually referred to as an "agent" or "proxy") can make binding choices on behalf of the patient (the "principal"), carrying out his or her wishes.

Note that two additional and critically powerful documents are a Last Will and Testament and a Trust. I mention them here for completeness. These legal documents are essential for the smoothest transfer of assets after death, but do not apply to events we experience during hospitalization.

The Option to Die in PEACE

The acronym PEACE expands to *Patient Ethical Alternative Care Elective*, an end-of-life reform initiative I developed during the writing of this book. PEACE, described in the chapter bearing its name, provides an alternative to what has become an American tradition: end of life under the influence of hospitalization. PEACE benefits all constituencies: (1) We the People, who choose to opt out of institutionalized dying; (2) providers who would rather focus on cure instead of dying and death, and (3) state and national policy makers and ethicists wrestling with questions of treatment resources, their costs, and future availability, (who can offer PEACE as a framework for their constituents to use to choose non-institutionalized dying, an arguably more humane and decidedly less expensive way to end one's life than in hospitals).

Non-institutionalized Dying

Non-institutionalized dying means dying in some place other than a hospital or nursing home, typically one's own home, some other private home, or at a hospice facility. This does not mean fighting death for weeks in a hospital before leaving (assuming one would still be in condition to leave) only to die several days later. It means avoiding a terminal hospitalization entirely, accepting one's dying, and doing so outside of the values, constraints, and angst that are virtually inseparable from dying in hospitals and related institutions.

Heroicism

At this writing, according to established dictionaries, "heroicism" is an un-word.[10] It is listed at www.unwords.com. Their definition is: *conduct or behavior relating to heroism; a lesser form of heroism.* How we understand heroic action, and when we believe it occurs, are key to our assessment of terminal hospitalization versus non-institutional dying (PEACE), and the latter's place in our lives. These thoughts are developed in the chapter "The Option to Die in PEACE."

Demise

According to the dictionary, *death and demise* are synonyms. In my mind and this book I make a distinction. Death for me is the *moment* of dying. Demise is the *process* of dying. Death lasts a moment; one's demise, or dying, can last weeks or months.[11] I don't expound on this elsewhere in the book, but know that this is generally my intention when I use the term *demise*.

Entity

An entity is the party across the table from you—in the abstract, an institution, but usually a person representing the institution. Hopefully an ally; at first, essentially a challenger. Some concepts apply to both hospitals and various financial or governmental institutions. When a concept is applicable to multiple institutions, I use the plural *"entities."*

Authentication

Authentication is proving to an entity, in response to its challenge, that (1) you are who you say you are and (2) you have the authority to engage in or direct your loved one's affairs according to the wording and scope of the document(s) that name you. Authentication requires that your loved one's Power Document(s) be in hand when you need them or, second best, that you can readily and quickly obtain them.

Preface | The Genesis of *Notes from the Waiting Room* ⁀⋀⋀⋀⋀

EVERYBODY WANTS TO GO TO HEAVEN; nobody wants to die to get there. In other words, being dead might not be so bad, but dying may be needlessly distressing, for both the patient and the family.

The Experiences Behind This Book

THIS BOOK IS NOT ABSTRACT. I have been involved with two deaths—those of my eighty-year-old mother, Ruth, in January 2004 and my eighty-four-year-old father, Mort, in May 2005. Both occurred during multi-week hospitalizations. Both were needlessly distressing.

I write from my involvement as a son who watched both parents die; as a personal representative (the designated power of attorney) for both health and financial matters, making critical decisions (including a life-and-death decision) on my father's behalf fifteen months after my mother's death; and as a trustee responsible for settling the family estate.

In both my parents' cases, their dying process was rife with unnecessary grief. I don't mean the natural grief that accompanies loss. I mean the needless grief we experience during health crises due to unforeseen patient-family languishing, unnecessary pain for our loved one, and requirements to make decisions we may not feel qualified to make—but which we must make nevertheless. The needless grief was not intrinsic to the situation (unexpected terminal illness) but was due to shocking extrinsic (external) causes.

I write as a layperson for lay people. I expose what causes much of the needless shock (and resulting grief) that can accompany any hospitalization and end-of-life experience.

I am not suggesting that grief be eliminated or is unnecessary. Grieving is part of loss, and healthy grieving is part of healing. In *Notes from the Waiting Room*, the focus is not on this natural grief but, rather, on how to prevent needless grief caused by shocking situations that need not occur.

Nor am I suggesting that every hospitalization past and future was and will be bad. It is possible to encounter truly caring providers. It is possible for communication to occur smoothly and for all to be right with your loved one's treatment. Such was not my family's experience, twice in a row, for the only parents I had.

Had my experience been limited to a single parent dying, I would not have proceeded with this book. I would have been just another family member among millions, griping about inexplicable and troubling experiences during a loved one's hospitalization or demise.

My second parent's demise included more of the same problems for the family, although different in their causes and details. The family was similarly impacted, even though we thought we had learned about hospitalization pitfalls, having lived through our mother's terminal hospitalization.

Since these events occurred in different institutions, neighboring cities, and fifteen months apart, a pattern seemed to emerge. As I considered our experiences, I set out to learn if they represented the norm.

Because I don't have medical initials after my name, I want to authenticate myself to you, brief you on my research, and introduce you to the array of professional helpers who ultimately confirmed my early theses (they where uninvolved with my later theses, specifically those informing The Option to Die in PEACE, although some have reviewed it).

Beginning Research

After my father's death and before starting this book, I engaged in two levels of research into these matters. The first level was the kind of research I believe most people might undertake when a need to know first arises: browsing bookstore shelves and searching the web using various search phrases entered into the popular online search engine Google and www.Amazon.com/books. This research yielded little I found of value. The searches located books on grieving, keepsake books (books of lists to make for survivors, one of which included a blank space for when the family home ought to get re-roofed), and various statistical analyses of hospitalizations. These do little to nothing to help us anticipate or deal with real-life events. They do zero to explain the nature of the environments in which we and our families are placed.

In an effort to make sense of our experiences and to determine if I was justified in my emerging view that our experiences were not isolated, I began interviewing professionals. Every healthcare professional I interviewed either generally or completely agreed with my findings. When one nurse and I discovered that both her mother and mine died in exactly the same horribly managed intensive care unit and that she, like my sister, Judy (a Newborn Intensive Care nurse), was reduced to utter ineffectuality there, I knew my family's story was not isolated.

The Unjuiced Story

At the same time as the preliminary investigations I embarked upon as a soul-searching quest during the summer of 2005, Judy authored an article to her nursing peers about her experience during the loss of our mother. After reading it, I felt impelled to offer my thoughts to this audience, adding to her clinical orientation my layperson's experience and perspective.

Shortly thereafter, Judy stimulated the interest of a local newspaper columnist in these matters. He wrote a column with enough inaccuracies and misconceptions that I had to write a follow-up. The columnist misinterpreted Judy's angst for hyperbole, saying she "juiced" her story. The word "juice" was the real hyperbole, one that required a response. The 750-word column I wrote in response summarized the first of my theses that have since become *Notes from the Waiting Room*: that absent or poor communication causes families in medical crisis to suffer extrinsic shocks that are exactly the opposite of what people need and expect under the circumstances (and which are the opposite of what actually constitutes *care*), and that these shocks have tremendous harmful effect during the most sensitive of times.

Key Background Reading and Exposure

During the several years it's taken to write *Notes from the Waiting Room*, I've unearthed a variety of interesting books on hospitalization and dying (see the annotated list under Suggested Reading). None of these has the focus that this book has, making *Notes from the Waiting Room* a light shining into a cavern heretofore closed from public view. The light will expose some skeletons, so we'll rattle their bones as we explore the place.

Two fields in particular have informed this book's evolution: medical ethics and medical anthropology,[12] neither of which I knew existed in 2004–2005. The work of two contributors to these fields especially informs my analysis and conclusions: the ethicist Diann Uustal and the medical anthropologist Sharon Kaufman. Their insights support fundamental aspects of the "Forecasting" and "The Option to Die in PEACE" chapters, respectively.

Additionally, the writings of patient rights and end-of-life rights advocates seem to be neighboring planets orbiting a sun around which my own independent conclusions have led me. Primary among these are Mark Meaney's *3 Secrets Hospitals Don't Want You to Know: How to Empower Patients*; Stephen Kiernan's *Last Rights: Rescuing End of Life from the Medical System*; and Tom Preston's *Patient-Directed Dying*.

Lastly, the work of healthcare policy analysis has been useful in providing a high-level glimpse into provision and cost society-wide. And although state and national policy makers do not offer guidance to individuals as to complying with proposed policy, *Notes from the Waiting Room* does.

Interviewees

A BOOK LIKE THIS OUGHT NOT BE COMPLETED at all without enough corroboration for you, the reader, to feel reasonably sure that the author's conclusions are meaningful beyond his own direct experience. Numerous people in varied roles graciously offered their time and experience, from which I gleaned that my conclusions are equally valid as a possibility for any American, anywhere in the country, dealing with hospitalization or end-of-life issues.

I interviewed various groups of people, who I list below in an order that I consider "bottom to top" in terms of their overall breadth of knowledge of a very complicated range of interlocking circumstances and disciplines. To be clear, each group's and individual's input has been of equal *value* throughout my research, thinking, and writing.

Plain Folk

For my information-gathering purposes, plain folk are people who have lived through and witnessed the demise of a loved one and shared their stories primarily as people rather than as professionals in the field. Although some report sporadic instances of kind and sensitive caring within the system, no one indicated that their experience was satisfactory overall.

Their stories acknowledge that the process of a loved one dying is full of intrinsic grief. Their focus while sharing their stories was on those times when the system required that they, as personal representatives, were required to intervene in order to obtain proper care for their loved one, or when they felt abused by individual treatment group members or by institutional practices and norms. Several plain folk are also long-time nurses, and their stories corroborated my sister's experiences. In recounting their stories, their grief was palpable.

Financial, Legal, and Funeral Professionals

These specialists' specific expertise helped identify and eradicate errors from the manuscript.[13]

Patient Liaisons

The patient liaisons I interviewed included a social worker, a registered nurse, and a representative of a medical subspecialty (bone ailments). From these people, I began learning about the challenges in their world and the constituencies they serve.

Nurses

I spent time with a range of nurses whose domains include the hospital floor, the emergency department, hospice, and consulting to the nursing profession. Some were interviewed as professionals and some as "plain folk" who had lost loved ones. One in particular, a friend and former emergency department manager who returned to nursing, lent valuable insight into ethical gray zones.

These beleaguered people educated me about the orientation of the nursing curriculum (to provide genuine care) and, by contrast, the sad realities in their hospital workplaces. Their workplace realities include (1) an executive management model[14] applied to nursing units and (2) narrowing job responsibilities used to extract maximum task performance from a shrinking nursing pool and their replacements. Their outlook ranges from an attitude of "march on" to utter demoralization. Some find that even their hospice work environment suffers from the maladies afflicting the hospital environment and that neither refuge nor respite is necessarily found there.

Doctors

The doctors I've been able to reach include a small set of private practice physicians who I engaged while in their office for periodic care, plus several ER[15] doctors.

Every doctor I encountered, both during my parents' demise and in conversation since, has generously given their time and attention, with the following exceptions: my father's primary physician during the latter part of his demise (she has taken my telephone calls since his passing) and both of his cardiologists (who cared for him in different regions during different times of his life), neither of whom responded to repeated messages during the year after his death.

One Emergency Department doc with whom I've had extended conversations has greatly expanded my awareness of the range of practical issues doctors must balance. Much of what he offered I agree with, and he has helped place my discussion of resuscitation in the context of an overarching treatment plan. However, in some of his views, I see reflections of systemic problems that, in my experience, impact us very negatively.

Hospital Administrators

I actually have not interviewed a career hospital administrator. Those I've contacted either directly or through intermediaries have refused to engage or be interviewed (by simply not responding). However, occasionally I have run across professionals from other groups who have previously been department or mid-level administrators or who have studied both business and healthcare. The sole high-level administrator I was able to talk to was the chair of an ethics committee (the context in which I contacted him), who also happened to be on the board of governors of a metropolitan healthcare system, currently including seven hospitals. He encouraged me to consider how society, technology, and hospitals intersect to form our current system, especially during end of life.

All of these people lent insight into what I believe to be administration attitudes. But without direct executive input, I cannot claim to directly know hospital administrators' views. I can only infer them based on my experiences and subsequent research. To me, their silence reflects precisely what they have to say to the public on these matters: nothing.

Ethics Committee Members

These people, almost always volunteers, help both families and practitioners sort out options. Their input introduced me to numerous ethical issues in the healthcare system and their sometimes-competing concerns and perspectives. They also introduced me to a group I consider the most surprising of resources: hospital chaplains and mission directors.

Chaplains and Mission Directors from Pastoral Care

Pastoral care personnel include hospital chaplains and, for those hospitals with formalized mission departments, mission directors. Mission directors will typically be found at religiously based hospitals, founded literally with or upon a sense of mission. They may direct the hospital chaplaincy and may or not be ordained ministers.

The pastoral care personnel I met with during my research have proven as a group to be the proverbial golden goose. All those I interviewed communicated kindness, wisdom, and generosity of spirit. More importantly, full-time chaplains are our point people, the gatekeepers to learning the nature and boundaries of the ethical resources in their institutions, plus how their institutions are organized. It was they who reinforced for me the important role filled by the emerging field of medical ethics.

Prior to my research, I had no interaction with chaplains in any setting. When describing my assessment of their value during hospitalization, some people have expressed surprise, citing their idea of chaplains as having a narrow religious focus while fulfilling a narrow religious role. While I can't vouch for every chaplain in every institution, those in forward-thinking hospitals have indicated no narrow sensibilities to me. While chaplains emerge from the clergy, their role is much broader, going well beyond ministry. Full-time hospital chaplains will know the lay of the ethical landscape in their hospitals. Thus, they emerge as primary go-to people, should we need help resolving deep healthcare problems. I explore the reasons why we might need such assistance in the forecasting chapter.

Medical/Clinical Ethicists

Ethicists proved to be the most personally rewarding individuals with whom I have conversed. Some have a nursing background, some a management background, and some an anthropology background. Some contributed significant amounts of time to my quest and greatly expanded my understanding of the countless issues that intersect during health crises. Those who consult to individuals are gifted, compassionate people with incisive minds and exquisite communication skills—combined attributes which I both bask in and aspire to. Their combination of clarity, warmth, and conviction when communicating is in and of itself healing. I found myself just wanting to hang out with them to soak in their goodness.

The Theses and Their Validation

NOTES FROM THE WAITING ROOM IS BASED UPON THREE THESES. The first two inform the book; the third arose from it.

My first thesis suggests two things. First, that hospitals do not provide care as lay people understand it; that, in fact, hospitals provide something else: bodily repair services. Second, that a two-part communication schism exists, with the bulk of hospital communications dedicated to convincing us they provide care, alongside a simultaneous absence of any meaningful communication addressing vital things patient-families need to know during their hospitalizations.

My second thesis is that absent or poor communication causes families in medical crisis to suffer extrinsic shocks, the opposite of what constitutes *care*, and that these shocks have a *profoundly* harmful effect on those families.

My third thesis, developed well into this project, postulates that the most effective way to manage a terminal hospitalization is to arrange not to have one.

As I interviewed and wrote, I kept waiting for healthcare professionals to tell me that one or more of my theses were wrong. No one did. To both my relief and dismay, that criticism has not been made. Rather, I have heard only the opposite message from them: that my conclusions were spot-on and an accurate, if regrettable, portrayal of the system writ large.

This is not to say that every hospitalization is problematic or that every demise includes systemic problems that impair families and magnify shock. Some hospitalizations may not evidence the problems my family encountered. However, professionals I interviewed confirm that the *nature* of situations I've experienced, examined, and describe represent a norm that could happen to anyone in any hospital anywhere in America.

Not About Blame

EVERYTHING I DESCRIBE IN THIS BOOK regarding lapses in patient care for my mother and father occurred as described. Although the litany of incidents may seem damning, my intention is not to damn, but rather to alert you to real and present dangers beyond those typically discussed in the media and within healthcare reformist websites (such as hospital-borne infections and surgical mistakes). The problems this book examines have not, to my knowledge, previously been analyzed nor codified.[16]

I won't damn a medical system that extended my father's life by nineteen years after his heart stopped cold, through the use of resuscitation, bypass surgery, and decades of chemical medicinal management.

(I call it *chemical life support*. If you're eating pills without which you will diminish and die, you're on life support).[17]

There's much that's right, good, and useful in the way hospitals apply medical science. Yet there's much that is also very wrong. Most of us would agree that much of what constitutes patient-family treatment in hospitals (misleadingly referred to as "care" by the healthcare field) is not very caring. What's wrong needlessly impacts us and our loved one in deeply intrusive ways at a time when we ought not be so impacted.

Writing without casting blame does not need to restrict analysis, reflection, and assigning responsibility. By learning how and why the system is what it is (including *our* part in it!), we can change essential and critical aspects of our experience during our loved ones' end days and their aftermath.

Writing without casting blame also does not mean writing without attitude. My family experienced situation after detrimental situation throughout two distinct hospitalizations in different institutions for differing medical problems. We feel that our best interests were not served in both cases and that, in each case, we were institutionally mistreated. My sister and I are not saints, and our emotional response to those events ranged from shock and bewilderment to anger—the echoes of which may occasionally arise in this book. I let them, because one of my intentions is to spur you on to action.

Dissatisfaction Clarified

When critiquing our medical treatment system, it's important to be clear about the basis of that criticism, especially what the critique is *not* based on.

Patient-family desires near or at end of life are personal and profound: a life is at stake. Here we must be careful: *Notes from the Waiting Room* does not emanate from any notion that either hospitalization killed my parents. They did not.

And since many circumstances that interest the media (and end up making law) include aspects of heroism, it's important to state that neither hospital denied heroic treatment. My mother's entire hospitalization occurred under heroic circumstances in the ICU. Ironically, the treatment denied to my father occurred under parameters that were decidedly non-heroic in nature. (During this book's conclusion, we will discuss the vital role our understanding of heroism plays regarding our loved one's end days. My viewpoint has changed; perhaps yours will, too.)

While I contend that in many ways, neither institution helped them, each elder was clearly in dire condition and hospitalized due to their individual cumulative frailty. This book's context is not that each parent died. Rather, it is the series of detrimental family experiences that made their passing more difficult and painful—more so than if our patient-family had received true care in the form of careful and compassionate guidance for managing our loved ones' hospitalizations and demise.

Disclaimers

I AM NOT A DOCTOR, NOR A LAWYER, NOR A FINANCIER. I do not claim expertise in all the medical ramifications and legal requirements surrounding end of life or other grave medical or legal events. None of what follows is intended, nor should it be construed as, medical or legal advice.

I offer my experiences along with some suggestions and insights in the hope that when you are faced with similar circumstances, you will already know what I had to learn moment by moment. When encountering circumstances such as those presented in this book, always seek and weigh the advice of medical, ethical, and legal professionals.

Throughout the book I write as if I were my father's sole personal representative. Actually, he designated my sister and I equivalent co-powers of attorney for both health and financial matters, each empowered to function alone if the other were unable or unavailable. We consulted and concurred on all matters, while dividing the many tasks that together comprise the management of a loved one's hospitalization (and also of estate settlement).

The assertions in this book are the result of my direct experiences. My conclusions result from examining those experiences and from subsequent research, which included corroboration by a range of medical professionals who I interviewed after my parents died. Some of those professionals have read the draft manuscript.

In the interest of refining future editions, I welcome input from readers, be you "plain folk" or those with medical, ethical, spiritual, legal, or financial expertise. Please send email to: Notes@AxiomAction.com.

For the Record: A Litany of Problems

Clinical and operational problems can arise in any hospitalization. At some point their number, frequency, and nature tips a scale and the cumulative patient-family experience turns negative.

The number of problematic events we experienced during my parents' end-of-life hospitalizations is lengthy. As you read the list you may think the balance of this book will focus on them. It will not.

I include the list below out of a sense that I ought to quantify our experiences. However, the problems cited are to our hospitalizations as bursting bubbles are to a pot of boiling water: symptoms, not cause. For water to boil, heat is required. For this range of events to transpire, some underlying element must be present from which the events emerge. Understanding and managing the underlying milieu will be our focus from the end of the list onward. For as perturbing as reading the events might be (and as distressing as living through them was), *Notes from the Waiting Room* addresses more fundamental issues that, when understood, will help you bring the entirety of a hospitalization or an end-of-life choice under your patient-family's conscious prior assent.

The following is a partial list of conditions we experienced during my mother's ICU stay. After arriving from out of state, Judy was there every day and was a direct participant in or witness to these events:

- A rounding doctor didn't notice or act on Ruth's low blood pressure until Judy pointed it out, despite it being visibly displayed on the bedside monitor.
- One day the respiratory therapist, in response to a family request to clear Ruth's mechanical ventilator tube, replied, "I can't stay at her bedside all day."
- Judy (a 35-year nursing veteran) was ushered out of the ICU for even minor procedures. She was denied the chance to touch her mother during the procedures—an act that would have been of

great therapeutic value to a daughter losing her mother (and per-haps also to the mother).

- ICU nurses didn't notice, act on, or advise the family about their patient's low 94° internal temperature; Judy brought this to their attention.
- After that, three-quarters of a day passed before receiving the doctor-ordered air mattress to help create a warm buffer.
- 24 hours later, the mattress was on the patient's bed but neither inflated nor plugged in.
- A number of rounding doctors routinely failed to address Mort, Ruth's husband. It appeared that they disliked that he was hard of hearing and that this slowed them down. They continued to ignore him in family conference despite the fact that he was obviously lucid, Mom's medical POA, and that Judy and I repeatedly told them to address him directly, even if she or I had asked the question being answered.[18] Eventually, I took to standing behind and slightly to the side of him to force practitioners talking to me to, on some level, talk to him.[19]
- The general noise level in the ICU was high. Unattended IV alarms went off, a supply closet door directly across the hall from our room was repeatedly left to slam, and nurses yelled to one another down the ICU hall about topics other than emergencies.
- Doctors routinely conducted critical care conversations directly over the patient (and quite loudly), despite widespread acceptance that unconscious patients can hear, and be troubled by what they hear in an environment they cannot engage with.
- Visitation hours began at 11 a.m. Since the doctors made their rounds between 7–9 a.m., conferencing with them became exceedingly difficult.
- When a death occurred in the facility, the ICU was locked down, shortening already brief visitation hours.
- Several times Judy had to intervene to prevent mislabelled IV drips from being attached to our mother (even if the label says it's the right substance, if the name on the container does not

exactly match the name of the patient, protocol says not to administer it).

- Equipment that dropped on the floor, instead of being disposed of, was picked up and put into immediate service on our loved one.
- For the most part, the nursing staff took an uncaring, cavalier attitude toward the family.
- After my mother was extubated and left to die, the nursing staff failed to call Judy when she was near death—despite Judy's explicit request to be kept closely advised of Mom's condition, despite the monitors that clearly indicated her withering vital signs, and despite the obvious mobility challenges Judy lived with as a result of her multiple sclerosis. The only reason Judy was alerted and present with Mom at her passing was that our cousins happened by around that time and called her. When Judy immediately called the ICU to inquire, they were brusque because it happened to be report time.

And as a final set of indignities:

- As death neared, there was no educating the family regarding what to expect.
- Family wishes were ignored. My sister had requested that Mom's monitoring alarms be turned off at the end, yet they were not. Finally, several minutes after Mom's passing, Judy shut down the machinery herself.[20]
- After Ruth flatlined and died, not one ICU staff member came to comfort Judy.

The following is a partial list of conditions we experienced at bedside during my father's hospitalization:

- Breaches of sterile technique in particular and hygiene in general.
- Lack of patient assistance in eating, resulting in multiple missed meals despite hunger.
- The effective withholding of liquids (drinking) due to the absence of assistance ingesting them (Dad's hands and arms were either

non-functional or hooked up to multiple IV drips).

- A technician carelessly ripping skin during a blood draw (which I consider abusive clinical treatment).
- Abusive treatment caused Dad by having a painfully-too-large catheter inserted into his penis (the RN acknowledged—after the fact—not having the right size at hand).
- Malpractice by a nurse who grabbed Dad's infected wrist after totally ignoring his presence and the nurse-sponsored signage above his bed warning against this action.
- Inadequate pain relief in both the hospital and hospice.
- During final decline in hospice, nurse failure to observe ongoing clinical distress such as copious fluids coming up through the mouth (i.e., drowning), requiring medical intervention to relieve.

FROM HERE FORWARD, *Notes from the Waiting Room* goes underneath, above, and around what I will here describe as the relative minutia of this litany. As grievous as these conditions were to experience, more important problems exist during hospitalization. My goal is to help you identify and understand why these sorts of events occur, discussing the best actions you can take to avoid similar events during your own patient-family hospitalization—to help you know in advance things you or a loved one may otherwise end up dying to know.

An Antidote to Profoundly Serious Problems

I OFFER THIS BOOK AS A GUIDE AND AS A SOLUTION for profoundly serious problems you may face during your loved one's hospitalization—especially if that hospitalization becomes an end-of-life event. Potential problems include, but are not limited to:

- Institutional practices that are questionable at best and detrimental at worst
- Stress and heartbreak associated with not getting information with which to make critical decisions in a timely manner
- Unquestioned ideas and expectations about what our medical system provides that shape our experience and add angst to it
- Last intimate opportunities with your loved one infringed upon or lost
- Bureaucratic runaround
- Unnecessary and harmful shock due to the above
- Enduring a terminal hospitalization because you don't know about or understand the alternatives.

This book will guide you to become qualified in advance, learning how to best represent your loved one by proactively and effectively dealing with "the system," and by offering an alternative to hospitalized dying and death.

Understanding "The System"

THE SYSTEM MAY BE PERSONAL OR IMPERSONAL. The system shows up as institutional and personal assumptions, hierarchies, values, ethics, procedures, rules, obstacles, omissions, and intersections of diverse interests. Contributing factors include:

- The patient's—your loved one's—mindset, values, and ethics
- Your own mindset, values, and ethics
- Your family dynamics, values, and ethics
- Our cultural milieu (societal and medical conventions)
- End-of-life medical entities and concerns—the curative, or allopathic, medical system comprised of doctors, nurses, hospitals, insurers; and hospice (a system providing end-of-life comfort, or palliative, care)
- Legal entities—the law itself, legal counsel, and governmental agencies
- Funeral and burial choices and entities
- Financial entities—banks, retirement fund companies, insurers, the government, and more mundane, day-to-day grantors of credit or service providers such as power, telephone, and internet providers (discussed in the companion book, *How to Efficiently Settle the Family Estate*).

During and after your loved one's death, you will likely deal with the system in its entirety (especially if the deceased is your second parent to die or your spouse). If you are the legally responsible person, you will encounter most or all the entities listed above as you grapple with each phase of your loved one's journey and the aftermath of their death.

Remember that *you and your family are part of the system*. This is true no matter what your viewpoint. To some extent, other entities in the system respond to your expectations and initiatives, your language and demeanor. To be sure, many of their activities occur due simply to how they function.

In any case, dealing with the entities during hospitalization and end-of-life times can be enormously challenging and stressful, because they rarely if ever tell you how they function. They rarely provide enough information for you to determine how to prevent things from happening that are not in your family's best interest.

In this book, I tell you how hospitals function and what you need to know in order to act in your family's best interest without the added stress and delay associated with learning on the spot, or the heartache of costly mistakes. I expose various surprising, baffling, aggravating, yet unfortunately common situations. I also share my research and conclusions regarding why things are the way they are.

Once you understand how and why hospitals function as they do, you can act preemptively to prevent unnecessary harm. If events you can't prevent do occur, you'll be better empowered to deal with them because you won't be totally taken by surprise. You may be dismayed, but you'll suffer little additional shock beyond the intrinsic shock of a serious hospitalization or death (which is plenty enough, isn't it?).

Assumptions

THIS BOOK ASSUMES A NUMBER OF THINGS that were true for me, but which may not be true for everybody. Some of these assumptions include the following:

- Your relationship with your loved one is fundamentally loving and healthy, and you want to do right by and for that person regarding health, life, and death.
- You are willing to expend the emotional and intellectual energy to involve yourself deeply in your loved one's care, and doing so falls within your value system.
- As a personal representative, you are intent on fulfilling your loved one's wishes, not your own or anyone else's.
- Your worldview and cultural norms allow you to take an active role in interpreting and managing your loved one's care, rather than handing off all responsibility to the medical treatment group.
- The hospitalization in question begins as, threatens to become, or in fact becomes a terminal hospitalization. (However, the

nature of hospitalization is the same no matter the seriousness of the ailment; bad turns can and do occur to those hospitalized for relatively trivial matters.)

- Your loved one's end days occur in the hospital or hospital-like environs, out-of-hospital options having been foreclosed. This could be due to failure to plan an out-of-hospital demise, failure to adhere to plans, or the breakdown of plans because of patient decline while in a hospital, which precludes their leaving.

- Your loved one becomes no longer capable of directing his or her own affairs; s/he is either totally unavailable or is accessible only for brief periods on a sporadic basis.

- During hospitalization you want to discover and absorb the most information you can as soon as you can with the goal of making informed decisions.

- Your relationship with your family is fundamentally healthy, and the family is either congruent in its outlook (e.g., in agreement about a treatment plan) or willing and able to become so.

- You have the time, financial reserves, and personal energy required to devote to managing these events.

Range, Focus, and Exclusions

This book details specific events that you may experience while your seriously ill loved one is in a hospital setting (especially if at their end of life).

As one examines end-of-life issues, a curious thing happens. The more you question, the more there is to question. A metaphor may better illustrate the complexity.

The Metaphorical Pond

You're familiar with the image of a stone dropped into still water and how the resulting wavelets, seen as concentric circles, get wider. They also disappear as they travel further from the impact point. By contrast, imagine that as the ripples spread out, instead of disappearing, the waves actually become bigger than they were at the point of impact. Now imagine an armload of boulders heaved into the water and all their waves growing and intersecting.

End-of-life issues are so complex that the further you travel from your initial point of inquiry, the larger and more interrelated the practical, ethical, systemic, and emotional waves become. Anybody standing on the shore of this metaphorical pond will get wet. Anyone navigating its waters will get emotionally, if not spiritually, tossed.

Therefore, it behooves us to acknowledge what this book addresses and what it does not.

Focus

There is a growing consensus in our nation that our current approach to healthcare matters ranges from terribly inadequate to completely broken.[21] I do not focus on how we got here, although I do address some history in passing. Rather, I write about what each of us is up against in the current medical treatment delivery system, as our parents or other loved ones die, and further into the future, when we and our contemporaries do.

The only rational alternative is to change the system—to the extent we can. This book offers two ways to change. First, by learning how the system works and how to best manage its workings. We can take actions to modify the system while we are in it, through our own approach, response, and behavior. Doing so can neutralize some of the worst transgressions. This inquiry occupies the majority of the book.

Second, by opting out of the system before we're subjected to its machinations. In chapter 9, "The Option to Die in PEACE," I propose a scenario that differs from institutionalized dying. The fundamental aspects of The Option to Die In PEACE are currently accessible to all citizens. PEACE has the potential to profoundly benefit us as individuals, as families, and as a society.

Although I focus on issues experienced during end-of-life situations, the discussions about Power Documents and resuscitation as well as the detailed examination of hospitalization apply equally to non-terminal hospitalizations. Because any hospitalization has the potential to turn deadly serious, if not terminal, much of this book may be valuable to anyone managing any hospitalization. However, end-of-life hospitalizations tend to devolve to multiple failures with numerous physicians on the case. These cases differ from single-disease hospital stays by predominantly younger patients, especially when the need arises to make ethical life-and-death decisions.

This book is for those who find themselves in these circumstances wherever they may occur in the United States. I focus on what any American family may encounter. My viewpoint is informed by my own particulars, where distant family members have the resources to buy a last-minute plane ticket to rush cross-country and stay away from home for some weeks (at the least), but who need to return to their own family, and get back to work to maintain a paycheck.

Exclusions

This book does not delve into issues specific to managing long-term care, whether a loved one lingers at their home, your home, a nursing home, special hospital, or within a hospice program. I have been told that similarities between hospitalizations and long-term care exist. If so, it's likely that what this book presents is applicable, in part, to long-term care situations. This is true especially if, during such lingering, your loved one is hospitalized once or more on a revolving-door basis, going back and forth between hospital and home—a situation that, if s/he wants to die a non-hospitalized death, represents a very real gamble.

I exclude a variety of topics that, although very important to the widest discussion, are outside of this book's focus. I do not delve into alternative healthcare modalities, philosophy, or religion. Nor do I attempt to dissect our national health insurance debacle. I cannot describe circumstances and situations that I have not experienced, been told about, or unearthed. I do not examine legal conundrums that could arise from hospitalizations. I do not suggest lawsuits. I have little to say about financial matters relating to hospitalization, as those I was involved with were paid by Medicare and we had no medical bills to reconcile. This book is not about grief or how to grieve. And I cannot speculate on hospitalization in foreign countries.

Nor, in this book, do I delve into the related complexities of closing a dying parent's home and settling the family estate, even though these tasks may overlap the time during which your second parent lies dying. (My companion eBook, *How to Efficiently Settle the Family Estate*, addresses many estate settlement tasks.)

A Zillion Variables

THERE ARE AS MANY WAYS to be sick, die, and manage the property left behind by a loved one as there are people, families, cultures, illnesses, caregivers, domiciles, municipalities, states, and estates. I can imagine a swarm of researchers compiling a lengthy reference detailing these many variables, each requiring updating as circumstances, institutions, and laws change. This book is not that tome.

Your circumstances undoubtedly will differ from mine. I cannot account for all the variables and do not promise to. However, the essential nature of hospitalization and end-of-life concerns remains constant. I touch on many essential aspects of managing end-of-life issues. You will learn various things that can make your exposure to and navigation of this phase of life easier—by providing you advance warning of events that may arise during grievously hard times and the knowledge to exercise control over those things that are controllable. As we continue, be nimble, willing to replace this or that personal detail of mine with your own.

Defining Families

A NOTE ABOUT FAMILIES IS IN ORDER. My family of origin remained intact, a traditional arrangement of married heterosexual people who together reared two children into adulthood. At the end, we adult children did what we could do to help aged parents leave this world.

Over my lifetime, societal boundaries around what may constitute a recognized family unit have loosened, at least to a place of open contention between citizens with differing ethics and viewpoints.

For this book's purposes, the common ground among people losing loved ones is the earthly bond that's about to be irreparably broken. Your imperiled loved one may not be a parent. And, any of us can designate non-family members as a medical or financial agent. Further, various ethnic cultures may subscribe to different ideas of inclusiveness or exclusiveness when it comes to medical decision-making.

My experience with these matters is in the context of my own family, and implicit in my presentation of them is the fact that they were my parents—unique relations with bonds spanning entire lifetimes, leaving an estate to settle upon their death. If your particulars differ from mine, remember: there are a zillion variables.

No matter how one defines family, the core quandaries associated with institutionalized dying are consistent.

Exposing the Unexposed

ESSENTIALLY, THIS BOOK IS AN EXPOSÉ. It exposes aspects of advance planning, hospitalization, and dying that, according to my experience and research, are not generally divulged to us before we need to grapple with them.

I learned the hard way, in real time, with detrimental effects to what was most important to us at the time—making the most of vanishing opportunities for communion with, and receiving direction from, my dying father (and conservation of my family's resources during estate settlement). Should you find yourself in the role of personal representative, I want you to have maximum breath and light, even as your loved one's breath and light fade and close. *Especially* because they fade and close.

I expose how the system works and what you may be likely to encounter throughout your dealings with it. These are vital issues that books by professionals usually gloss over—issues that may make a critical difference at a crucial moment for your loved one and yourself.

Several Unexpectedly Big Topics

IN ADDITION TO THE POTPOURRI OF EVERYDAY HOSPITAL ISSUES, several topics are so big that I devote entire chapters to them.

These include the tightly intertwined issues of communication and care in the hospital setting, the related issues of forecasting and obtaining ethical support, and a top-to-bottom examination of resuscitation. In my experience, understanding these topics—more importantly, understanding their *consequences*—comprise the foundation upon which we can effectively manage all the other important issues that arise during hospitalization. Conversely, failing to understand these topics and their internal relationships leaves us open to the most disruptive and painful experiences that can possibly occur during a loved one's hospitalization and/or end days.

Emotional Understanding and the Urgency to Act

MY INTENTION IS THAT YOU UNDERSTAND the nature of hospital deficiencies both intellectually and emotionally. Other books discussing how to successfully navigate hospitalizations, valuable as they are, seem to ignore or fail to communicate an emotional imperative to act. Most are written by doctors (including those who have finally experienced the system as patients or as a personal representative to a hospitalized spouse), some are written by journalists, but only a very few by a layperson such as myself. While doctors' insider knowledge is valuable, their offerings fail to acknowledge the emotional challenges families face when forced to make impossible choices—or worse, are abandoned by the system as they do so.

A case in point is Do Not Resuscitate orders. Books by medical professionals typically provide scant discussion, if any, regarding resuscitation matters. But it's a huge topic with enormous ramifications. *Notes from the Waiting Room* includes a thorough examination of all aspects of resuscitation as manifested both in and out of hospitals: "The Complete Do-Not-Resuscitate Conversation."

Despite learning from many books' insights and authoritative presentations, I tend not to feel compelled to act as a result of reading them. I hope that this book's emotional content, interspersed with analysis and information, will serve you. I hope to instill in you a visceral understanding of what you stand to lose by not acting versus what you can gain by becoming the most effective personal representative that you can possibly be. I hope to empower you to take effective action at every moment that doing so will benefit your patient-family. Your choice in any moment may well resonate throughout your lifetime. If I save you a moment's heartache or its lingering echoes, this book will have succeeded.

SECTION 1 | **EFFECTIVELY REPRESENT YOUR LOVED ONE**

N O MATTER WHAT YOUR LOVED ONE IS HOSPITALIZED FOR, s/he is at significant additional risk without your effective personal representation.

Effective means that you know how to function in the role of personal representative, and that you do so in ways that make a positive difference in your patient-family's experience and outcome.

Effectiveness in this role also requires that a protective legal framework be established around your patient-family by executing a series of legal forms. Without the suite of five legal documents I call "Power Documents," you run a real chance of the system freezing you out of decision-making. Will it? Who knows—but why place yourself at such a risk?

Thus, we begin with two chapters discussing "front-end" matters.

Chapter 1, "Be An Effective Personal Representative," examines how to function as a personal representative in a uniquely challenging environment, offering numerous steps you can take to ensure that you do.

Chapter 2, "Making Effective Declarations: The Essential Power Documents," presents the legal requirements you must meet in order to be recognized as your loved one's legal and authoritative voice, without which you and your loved one could be rendered powerless.

If you feel particularly eager to delve directly into the everyday situations encountered during hospitalization or the weightier aspects of whether even to go, sections two and three await you. Chapters 5 through 10 discuss progressively weightier, alarming situations. Should you skip to them, I strongly urge you to return here and read section 1. Understanding what effective personal representation entails and constructing a secure legal framework around your family's affairs are your patient-family's bedrock foundations, and the only aspects of hospitalization that are under your sole control.

1 | Be an Effective Personal Representative

"*B*ART, DID YOU TURN THE COMPUTER OFF?" *This was one of the few questions my father asked me during his terminal hospitalization. I lied: "Yeah, Dad, I did."*

My father continued moving his uninfected arm over his abdomen in a strange motion I'd come to recognize but not yet understand. "Good, it was doing this to me."

Mort ranked among the most intelligent one percent of the population, a member of Intertel, an international group of the world's smartest people. I knew him as always lucid, with a penetrating mind. His diseases were physical, not mental. I was not prepared for, and didn't immediately comprehend, his delusional comments.

The night I arrived at his hospital bedside in dismay, internal agitation, and a son's diminutive role, I failed to ask questions. I wasn't expecting to encounter symptoms associated with the possible onset of death—although that was exactly what I was encountering, even though I didn't recognize them at the time.

During his last twenty years, Dad had endured a number of serious hospitalizations (some of which saved and added decades to his life), and we believed him when he subsequently said he'd engage in no more. Now he was hospitalized again, but this time he was physically helpless and debilitated.

After learning that Dad was crying in his hospital room (the call came from our cousins, not from hospital staff), my sister Judy had immediately flown there, preceding me by six days. This was a man who didn't cry and who had been supremely logical all of his life. He would never have accused his home computer of messing with his insides, not even in jest. This sort of illogic was outside his worldview. He had spent the first half of his working years as an electrical engineer, with a profound respect for the design, manufacture, use, and maintenance of machines.[22]

The moment I arrived in his hospital room, he called a "meeting" to order and made a declaration. "Sometimes you have to shit or get off the pot. I have decided to shit."

I interpreted Dad's crude metaphor as a defense mechanism against the seriousness of his predicament. When facing severe physical breakdown, speaking plainly can be very very difficult, for plain talk is a stark and honest mirror. As I recall, Dad's figure of speech was the only statement he was able to make that night before lapsing into unconsciousness. I was too slow to ask him exactly what he meant by it and what his intentions were, given his debilitated condition and prior vehemence against any further hospitalization.

I had good excuses to have failed at this moment. I was fresh off a hastily arranged, ten-hour journey that had taken me through three airports. My father was unexpectedly in dire condition, and my sister was almost as debilitated as he, due to the stress associated with managing his hospitalization plus her own multiple sclerosis.

I knew I'd be assuming a pivotal role, yet this unexpected "meeting" and pronouncement shook me. This was intrinsic shock, trauma that logically results from the situation.

In those first moments, that first night, I had not yet

flipped the mental switch to become Dad's personal representative. I was the son of a man who had always been in charge and who had cheerfully driven himself to the hospital just a few days ago, believing the cardiac stress tests were...

I don't know what he believed, but during our prior conversations, I was under the impression the hospital stay was a safety precaution due to his advanced years and complex medical condition.

As the next weeks unfolded, it turned out that I functioned in dual roles: adult child and designated personal representative. I could never quite ask my father the sort of hard questions I had no problem asking his physicians (when I could think to ask them). This failure damaged me more than him...or so I like to think.

FOR THOSE IN ACUTE NEED OR CRISIS

PERSONAL REPRESENTATIVES AGREE TO SERVE their loved one in one or two specific legal relationships that are recognized by people and institutions in the medical, financial, and legal realms. Their recognition requires that legal documents be drafted IN ADVANCE, signed (with witnesses), and most important, presented to the people and institutions caring for your loved one and their property.

Other terms for personal representative include surrogate, proxy, agent, and advocate. From a layperson's perspective, none adequately connote your relationship to and role in support of your loved one. Plus, "advocate" is used more frequently to refer to some third party rather than the agent named in a Medical Power of Attorney (presumably that's you). No matter the label, you act in your loved one's stead, and you advocate for his or her interests.

EFFECTIVE PERSONAL REPRESENTATION IS REQUIRED in order to protect the well-being of your hospitalized loved one and to expedite property transfer from the estate to its heirs should your loved one die.

Effective personal representatives extend their loved one's desires, not their own. As a personal representative, you will actively question everything and everyone (including your loved one) in order to reach decisions -- sometimes difficult ones. You have authority and will use it (wallflowers need not apply, or need to quickly gain comfort stepping away from the wall). You dedicate yourself to the demands of the role, including long hours every day spent waiting, questioning, documenting, consulting, and doing countless other tasks.

You do all of this because, in general, you won't otherwise learn what you need to know in advance, to protect your loved one and best manage their case.

Somehow, you manage also to TAKE CARE OF YOURSELF.

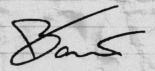

What is a Personal Representative?

WHEN MANAGING A LOVED ONE'S AFFAIRS as a personal representative, two distinct realms exist: the medical and the financial. These affairs are carried out by persons functioning as the Medical Durable Power of Attorney and Property Durable Power of Attorney. For our conversation, that means you. The Medical POA controls healthcare decisions, and the Property POA controls transactional decisions ("transactional" means that you can transact business on behalf of the person who designated you as their property power of attorney).

The medical personal representative is a formal position with distinct and sobering legal powers. Your loved one must have designated you to act as his or her personal representative by filling out ("executing") a document titled Medical Durable Power of Attorney[23]. Additionally, your loved one must be incapable of acting or communicating on their own behalf before you can intervene with legal authority to direct their treatment.[24] "Directing their treatment" means taking over fundamental decision-making, which may include making life-and-death decisions. Caregivers, administrators, and authorities must acknowledge your authority and act according to your direction—insofar as their own professional responsibilities, legal requirements, and ethics allow. What becomes most problematic is when their ethics or the requirements around their roles come into conflict with your family's values and wishes.

The "Effectively Manage Hospitalization" section demonstrates how ethical differences may play out by detailing several critical ethical problems my family encountered and their detrimental effect on us.

More importantly, I'll describe how you can learn in advance what, if any, hospital resources are available to help you resolve ethical conundrums. If the institutional resources exist and the individuals involved are mature and empowered, you can draw upon compassionate expertise to help explore and resolve differences within your own mind and heart, between family members, and between your family and the treatment group.

Of equal or greater importance on a day-to-day basis, I'll describe what steps to take to avoid experiencing the damaging emotional shock of unanticipated circumstances that tend to compound ethical conundrums.

Why is a Personal Representative Needed in Hospitals Today?

NO ONE LOOKS AFTER YOUR INTERESTS LIKE YOU DO. Staff people do not have the time, orientation, or professionalism to adequately take on this task. A personal representative is needed because hospitals do not provide care in the way we as laypersons understand care. You may already have encountered reports in the media cautioning us about how hyper vigilant we must be during hospitalizations. They're not exaggerated, and the situation is poised to worsen in the coming decades due to the dwindling number of nurses and growing number of aging citizens who will soon require more treatment.

What Makes a Personal Representative Effective?

WHEN REPRESENTING A LOVED ONE WHO IS VULNERABLE and unable to represent him- or herself, being effective is truly important. This is a profound responsibility at a time with grave stakes. Let's examine exactly what effective personal representation entails.

You Champion Your Loved One's Wishes

A key aspect of acting effectively as someone's Medical Power of Attorney is that *you learn, understand, and champion* (commit to fulfilling) *that person's wishes.* In other words, you are your loved one's advocate.

Presumably you've been selected and agreed to serve because your outlook is congruent with your loved one's outlook. During my father's demise, I said, "I am not here to usurp my dad's authority. I am here to extend it." This was the case for my family, and I hope it's true for yours. If not, you've got a serious additional level of involvement to contend with, one that this book does not address beyond mentioning it here.

Being a personal representative differs from being one of several concerned family members in conference. A family in conference looks inward together, with varying degrees of authority dispersed among family members. As personal representative, you possess explicit legal (and ethical) authority, which you will direct outward to the treatment group and, if necessary, beyond.

You Use Your Authority

As an effective personal representative, you assume and use the authority legally granted to you by your loved one. An important distinction: having authority and using it are two different things. Your ability to advocate on your loved one's behalf may require that you direct (or redirect) the treatment group—sometimes gently, other times forcefully.

Based on my experiences during each of my parents' deaths, you, as personal representative, will need to oversee, intervene, correct, and otherwise actively involve yourself in your loved one's treatment. Doing so effectively requires that you understand why and how things happen (or don't happen) in the hospital setting. Since you most likely can't rely on hospital staff to explain what you *really* need to know, Section 2, "Effectively Manage Hospitalization" communicates what I believe all hospitals and providers should be required to convey.

It is important to take proactive steps in support of your loved one's interest. Wallflowers cannot prevent wrongs from occurring or right wrongs after they've occurred. You may use your authority with grace, equanimity, or anger by turns. But use it you must, else your loved one will be at greater risk. If you feel you cannot wield this authority, it's better to decline its responsibility in the first place.

The Medical Durable Power of Attorney document must be submitted to an institution in order for those who practice there to recognize you as a patient's personal representative. (We'll review the necessary legal documents in the next chapter, "The Essential Power Documents.") As a practical matter, doctors seem by default to acknowledge family members in a hierarchical order as having authority to speak for a loved one and to direct their treatment, assuming the patient cannot do so personally. That was my experience, where two adult children were the patient's entire nuclear family, and my research reading corroborated it. In large families with, for instance, several elder siblings and many adult children, I do not know how doctors establish the hierarchy.[25] For large families, it becomes all the more important for people to (1) make their wishes clearly known throughout the family circle and (2) to execute an advance directive and a Medical Power of Attorney designating their personal representative.

Financial representation differs from medical representation; the two realms are totally separated, although they begin similarly. Your loved one designates his/her financial personal representative by executing the Property Durable Power of Attorney[26] document. If you're designated and your loved one is incapable of acting on their own, you can transact business on their behalf.

You Become a "Professional" Question-asker

Another characteristic of an effective personal representative is no-holds-barred questioning. It's counterproductive to wield authority in the absence of sufficient information. Much of your effort as personal representative may involve tracking down, obtaining, interpreting, conveying, assessing, and even agonizing over medical information. There's only one way to get it and gain an understanding of it: ask everything of everyone, again and again.

You Ask Everything of Everyone, Again and Again

The notion of asking questions continually, relentlessly, assumes a lot of you, namely that you want to involve yourself deeply in your loved one's care in order to best understand the treatment plan, options, and decision points. This requires you to become what I call a professional question-asker.

As a professional question-asker, *the only wrong questions are the ones you don't ask*—again and again, of many different people.

There are vital reasons for asking questions relentlessly and repetitively during a medical crisis or hospitalization. The environment is foreign. Your loved one's well-being, perhaps life, is at stake. The treatment plan has to be developed and carried out, and it is subject to change. In spite of long waits, decisions will need be made and acted upon, some of them on very short notice (unless they've been forecast, the absence of which is a serious problem we'll discuss further on). Medical mistakes and omissions occur, so the more you become familiar with your loved one's treatment, the more you can accurately monitor it.

For some of us, asking questions comes easy. For some, it can be excruciatingly hard. I'm in the former group, for several reasons. First and foremost, it's how I learn. I like my world my way, and I end up engaged in lots of projects, making new things with unfamiliar materials and techniques. I ask many questions, often the same questions, of multiple people to triangulate the answers. I find that asking questions repeatedly invariably results in the best information rising to the top, as I cross-reference the answers through a process of repetition, clarification, and verification. And as a writer, part of my job description is "professional question-asker."

At the end of this chapter, I offer some suggestions to help you become a proficient question-asker. And I'll reinforce this role at the end of each succeeding chapter.

You Look Ahead, asking "What if?"

This book exists because I've witnessed and experienced severe emotional shocks due to mismanaged or absent communication involving hospitalization and financial events. The communication deficiency emanates from medical and financial institutions' failures to anticipate the questions that matter most to people and failing to answer them up front.

Anticipation is a quality that you, as a professional question-asker, want to exercise. The basic questions to pose when projecting into the future are "and then what?" and "what if?" When it comes to medical matters during hospitalization, you will find it's better to learn about your loved one's condition, prognosis, and trajectory sooner rather than later. Why? Because you and your family will have more time to consider how you want to respond to the major possibilities in advance of their occurring.

I acknowledge my bias for informed involvement. It stems from a desire for control. That desire is based on our experiencing numerous unnecessary shocks during each of my parents' hospitalizations and as I settled the family estate. From these experiences comes my assessment that effective personal representation requires a tenacious personal representative.

Interestingly, this is verified time and again by doctors who have learned through their experience as patients or personal representatives and subsequently recommend that a personal representative stick like glue to their hospitalized loved one, staying with them 24/7 to oversee treatment and act on their behalf.

Not all groups, families, or individuals want to know. In some eastern cultures, the family does not involve an ill loved one in medical decision-making. According to one ethicist with whom I spoke, the family seeks to shield their loved one from projections, debates, and decisions. These cultural values may be more predominant in immigrants or first-generation Americans.

No matter where one's cultural roots take hold, and for whatever reasons, some mainstream American individuals or families may not want to involve themselves deeply in patient care. They may prefer to give the doctors and establishment free rein to perform as best they see fit.

This book assumes that you have encountered institutional and personal errors throughout your life. These errors have ranged from picayune to maddening, and they always cost time, energy, and money. During a loved one's hospitalization, much more is at risk. The risks are many orders of magnitude larger than haggling about last month's cell phone bill.

At its most demanding, the question-asker's role requires that you become like a periscope, looking around corners at all possibilities and asking the party with whom you are dealing, "what if this?" and "what if that?" "What will you do if ABC?" and "what do you need from me, and when, if XYZ?" "If this were to happen, then what? If that were to happen, then what?" If that party is a doctor, be sure to add, "What outcome do you expect if we follow your recommended course of treatment?"

Jazz musicians say that there are no wrong notes, only wrong connections. Unstated is the fact that you have to pick up an instrument and play in order to make any connections, right or wrong. I can't blow this horn loud or long enough: the only wrong questions are unasked questions, because without answers to questions, you can't make connections. What you don't know can and may actually hurt you, your loved one, and your family. You need foreknowledge to make effective life-and-death, health-and-wealth decisions.

You Ask Direct Questions of Your Loved One
Before it's Too Late to Get Their Answers

Asking direct questions of your loved one about what they want for their care is among the most important jobs you have. And one of the most difficult.

Life-and-death matters require clear communication. In these moments, evasion, beating around the bush due to discomfort, and the use of innuendo or metaphor serve no one. If you think your loved one is dying or may die, and you're unsure of their desires, ask before it's too late. The alternative is that you, as personal representative, will be making some very tough decisions. (See "Death Looks Like This" for descriptions of common indicators of possible impending death. If you don't recognize such signs, you will lose precious opportunities to interact with your loved one while s/he is still able to interact with you.)

I know how hard asking direct life-and-death questions of a loved one can be. I failed at it. My father became unavailable without my having asked him what he wanted as he moved closer to a death that, maybe, possibly, could have been postponed for a meaningful period of time without heroic intervention. My sister and I agonized during a weekend about the life-and-death decision we had no option but to make ourselves.

It may not seem like it in the abstract, but ultimately making a decision that hastens someone's death is harder than asking your loved one to decide that for him- or herself. If you need guidance, seek out a chaplain or ethicist who's skilled in these most delicate of matters. I'll discuss these individuals' great importance and value in the forecasting chapter.

You Document Every Conversation, Observation, and Action

Effective personal representation requires that someone in the attending family record every conversation, observation, treatment, and action in a notebook dedicated to this purpose. Consider this record a parallel to the record the hospital maintains on your loved one (the *chart* or medical record for this particular hospitalization). In it, log the date and time, location, name and title or role of the person with whom you're consulting. (Ask, for instance, "Are you a registered nurse or a technician?")

For each event write down *what, when, why, who, where, what outcome, what/when next.* Leave space under each entry to add questions that subsequently arise.

One reason is simple: The medical world is a highly technical place, and providers speak a specialized language. Unless you write things down, you will forget. What you write and review will assuredly stimulate further questions as events proceed. And your own record, the personal "chart" that you make, will be written by and for you, so it may be more understandable than the hospital chart written by and for doctors and nurses.

Another reason for keeping your own chart is that, under certain circumstances, you can be denied access to your loved one's hospital chart. For instance, without a legally binding Medical Power of Attorney document, and a HIPAA[27] release that's completely independent of any other circumstances, the hospital is not required to allow you access to the chart, no matter what your relationship to your loved one is, *even if you're the spouse.*[28]

Over time, you'll get to choose how much of the lingo you want to use when conversing with the treatment group. The upside of using the treatment group's language is that you may facilitate a conversation by indicating you understand and are comfortable with at least some terminology. The downside is that using even a little may cause some people to assume you know more than you do. This would require you to humbly ask for certain statements to be repeated in lay terms. This is OK; the docs are used to it. In this realm, be brave! This is the time and place to leave self-consciousness behind. The benefits are more than worth any discomfort, and the only way to acquire facility with a new language is to use it.

If the rigor of maintaining a chart is daunting, consider keeping a journal. Journaling differs from charting in that the former reflects one's private thinking and charting documents things that occur and are said. During hospitalizations, journaling will probably record at least some of what's occurred and will likely stimulate questions to pose to the treatment group.

Another option is to use a hand-held tape recorder or digital voice recorder. A digital voice recorder is a tiny device you can slip into your pocket or purse (the one I used for interviews while researching this book measures less than 5" x 1.5" x 1"). They range in price, starting from about $40 (I bought a $150 model). Keep spare batteries with you. Better yet, use lithium cells; they'll probably power your recorder every time you need it.

The benefit to voice recorders is that you can play back conversations to verify what was said (versus what you thought you heard). Downsides include the fact that the device is itself a gadget you need to learn how to use correctly, and the recorded conversations ought to be (1) backed up to a computer and/or CD and (2) transcribed into the notebook anyway, as browsing the notebook is actually the more efficient data retrieval method (unless you have the tools and technical savvy to translate from speech to text and a computer you keep with you at all times).

Another potential downside regards human relations. I didn't have a digital recorder in the hospital, so I don't know how doctors, nurses, and administrators would respond to having their conversations with the patient-family recorded verbatim. Some might be comfortable; others might view a desire to record as antagonistic.

Another piece of technology that will help if you have a cell phone is a headset, either wired or wireless, preferably with voice-activated dialing, a real efficiency booster. The ability to make and field calls hands-free is extremely beneficial. (When in the hospital, you'll have to decide for yourself whether or not to abide by the signs asking you to keep the cell phone turned off.[29])

You Surrender to the Demands of Time

In the "Effectively Manage Hospitalization" section I discuss the nature of what I call *hospital time*, that strange, other time zone. Consider my family's scenario as a baseline, where for two to four weeks you're halfway across the country, with a home, job, and life to return to. You have limited vacation time and sick leave. Your financial resources have limits. You're with your dying second parent, and you are both the Medical and Durable Power of Attorney.

Every item that pops up as a to-do needs to be done ASAP. By "done"

I mean *begun*. Because, as I learned, there are always delays in completing to-dos, and the time it takes to accomplish a to-do item will invariably stretch.

If you have unlimited time to remain away from home or the luxury of traveling back and forth to deal with post-death asset transactions, you might not have to hop on each and every new to-do item like a shooter at a carnival target game. But if you must return home on a given date, be aware that some issues require lead time to complete before that date.

It's a lot of work. I didn't do it alone; my sister shared both roles of Medical and Durable Power of Attorney with me. She focused on medical matters due to her clinical knowledge and physical limitations of multiple sclerosis, and I focused on most of the rest: research, arrangements, and running around dealing with estate settlement matters, even as my father lay dying. We conferred on managing Dad's hospitalization, with me traveling the halls when implementing our decisions required that I find some provider, since my mobility was not impaired and hers was.

Prepare for long days populating long weeks. I recall going about ten days straight, from early morning to midnight, before taking a few hours off for a massage and to sit by a lake for an hour doing nothing before returning to my dual representative roles. I don't recommend such a rigorous regimen for most people under these circumstances.

You Take Care of Your Own Well-Being

Acting as a loved one's personal representative during grievous times is a walk-on role for most of us, one for which there are no rehearsals. And no second takes. The role's unique stressors and demands equate to a condition I call a *crucible*: a place of severe test or trial.

Caregiver stress has a name: *caregiver stress syndrome*. Reformists are currently trying to get this condition clinically recognized by the medical establishment.

Severity takes its toll, and the last thing you need is to make yourself sick or ineffective. So, somehow, take care of your own needs and well-being, too. Doing so is as important as taking care of your loved one.

Why is Effective Personal Representation Important?

It's Unusual to be Told What May Lay Ahead

Among medical ethicists, sharing with the patient and family what may lay ahead is called *forecasting*. Forecasting is different from the presentation of a treatment plan and its prognosis, although the best treatment plans include forecasting.

You'll know forecasting if you get it. And you'll know if you don't get it, because you'll feel very uncertain about the existence of various branches of a treatment plan, their potential outcomes, target dates for key procedures and choice points requiring decisions, and other possible outcomes. In fact, they'll appear out of the blue, and you'll most likely reel in shock from their impact.

Medical professionals and representatives of governmental and financial entities understand that they are responsible to your loved one through you. In our dealings with many of them, we found most individuals to be courteous and ready to engage—providing we prompted them for information.

In the hospital environment, in my family's experience during both end-of-life situations, the norm was "don't ask, don't tell." If we didn't ask for information, there was no guarantee it would be offered. I don't know if this was intentional, a result of understaffing, or for some other reason such as discontinuity of care (topics I address in the "Effectively Manage Hospitalization" section). I tend to think that in our cases, the reason was the underlying institutional milieu in the region (south Florida). However, industry professionals told me multiple times while researching this book that despite south Florida's reputation as "ten years behind the times" in terms of hospital customer orientation and service, the problems we experienced are more or less the norm in any hospital, anywhere in the United States.

Despite the apparent reluctance to communicate that we experienced, medical personnel are ethically required to answer your questions fully, according to the American Hospital Association's Patient's Bill of Rights.

When it comes to ongoing, comprehensive communication about

your loved one's condition, prognosis, and your role as a personal representative in the hospital, assume nothing. Ask for explanations for everything, and keep asking until you are sure your questions have been completely answered and that you understand the answers. Ask the same questions of multiple practitioners. Aside from triangulation, you never know what tidbit of information may be offered that leads to another important clarification, resource, or avenue of inquiry.

Don't be put off by the idea of asking what-if questions. I've found two reasons for posing them: first, by extending a conversation, interesting and even vital new information may emerge. Second, the conversation may help you see a little further into one potential future, giving you advance insight into, and preparedness for, what could be the next phase of decision-making. In other words, by asking what-if questions, you are helping the treatment group provide your family with forecasting.

It's important, however, to ask questions of the right people. As an example, it is reasonable to ask administrative questions of a hospital admissions clerk as well as a physician practicing in the facility. It would be unreasonable to ask the clerk questions about a loved one's treatment plan, but it would be reasonable to ask the nursing staff those questions, in addition to the attending physicians.

During hospitalization, the challenge is to manage risk. After death, the concern is minimizing the already gargantuan amount of time even simple property disposition and estate settlement require. When this occurs out of state and you need to return home sooner than later, decisions may need to be made quickly. If you are local, or have already returned home, it becomes a matter of efficiency, where inefficiency can drain massive amounts of your time.

Without Representation There is an Increased Risk of Damage

The most important reason that effective personal representation is important is that without it, damage may occur to your family. This is not to induce fear or guilt; it's just the logical outcome of poor information transfer or insufficient patient oversight.

There are several ways to learn. One way is in advance. That's called "school". Another way is on the spur of the moment. That's called the "school of hard knocks." "Hard knocks" is an understatement, considering the difficulties this book describes.

Spur-of-the-moment medical revelations (surprise informational hard knocks) received during serious hospitalization disrupt your equilibrium. They land like an emotional bomb in your midst. They induce anxiety. They take a toll on your family, and the more physically compromised a family member is, the tougher that toll is to endure and witness. I watched my then eighty-three-year-old father take in and physically recoil from extrinsic emotional shocks at my dying mother's bedside because of things that shouldn't have happened and could have easily been avoided had the system oriented itself toward careful family treatment.

Our family came together. Although Dad was my mother's medical agent, in a way my sister and I functioned as Dad's agent. No one expected Dad to be standing at his dying wife's bedside. For decades, our family expected the reverse; that Mom would outlive Dad. His shock reduced his agility. Judy and I were mentally quicker, so we essentially took on the role of dual representatives (this foreshadowed our legal role as co-medical agents during Dad's demise fifteen months later). Judy and I functioned as professional question-askers.

How to Get Comfortable in the Role of Question-Asker

HOW DO YOU BECOME A PROFESSIONAL QUESTION-ASKER if you're uncomfortable asking questions? Maybe you're introverted, extremely trusting, uncomfortable challenging authority, or your cultural background precludes assuming a questioning role.

While postulating psychological reasons for discomfort in the role of question-asker is beyond my expertise, I can offer the following suggestions to overcome hesitation:

- Make a list of things you want to know.
- Ask small questions first.
- Question people with less authority before questioning those with more authority (example: admissions clerk before physician).

- Ask questions of the appropriate person. For instance, you might ask an admissions clerk what they do with your elderly parent's DNR form, and save for the physicians questions regarding how the treatment group will behave toward your loved one given their DNR status.

- Try to stay as neutral as possible. People generally respond well to innocent inquisitiveness.

- Be clear about why you need to know what you're asking for, and if need be, share your reasons for needing to know. (Hint: since we don't know what we don't know, asking questions simply to learn if what we hear matters to us is a perfectly good reason.)

- Ask questions to which you already know the answer (or think you know the answer). This is a proven technique to assess the knowledge or perspective of the person who you are questioning.

- Be persistent until you get an answer and understand it.

- *Remember that your loved one's comfort, return to health, perhaps their life may well depend upon your active intervention.*

And what about the specter of appearing dumb or ignorant? Guess what? The medical world is complex. The people serving your patient-family have clinical expertise. They may not know everything, but they are deeply trained and experienced. Take advantage of your proximity to them every day you're in their workplace and at your loved one's hospital bedside. If they don't have an answer for you, ask them either to obtain it or advise you how to obtain it.

Give yourself permission. *You* are the only person with the legitimate authority to allow or restrict your own question asking.

This Book is the Place to Start Asking Questions

If you're unsure or uncomfortable asking questions, this book can help get you started. What questions arise for you throughout our conversation? By the end of each chapter, have those questions been answered? If not, how will you get them answered? I'll prompt you by asking these questions as we move from chapter to chapter throughout this book. This chapter's prompt appears immediately below.

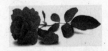

Personal Representative Recap: What You Can Do

If your loved one is hospitalized, document everything throughout each day and night. Maintain notes (your personal "chart") or keep a journal.

Be an effective question-asker! *Start now.* Has this chapter answered all your questions about:

- What is a personal representative?
- Why is a personal representative required?
- What makes a personal representative effective?
- Why is being an effective personal representative important?
- What might happen if I'm not an effective personal representative?
- What can I do to gain comfort as a relentless question-asker?

If you do not have all the information you need, write your questions down. How will you get them answered? Reread this chapter? Internet research? Library research? Consulting with family and friends? A phone call to a professional or organization? Go online or pick up the phone book, find a likely contact, and send the email or place the call.

2 | Making Effective Declarations: The Essential Power Documents

S PRING WINDSURFING ON LAGUNA MADRE *between South Padre Island and Port Isabel, Texas is extraordinary. During April 2005, the sailing was fast and totally engaging. Strong, steady wind over warm, shallow water contributed to Padre's ideal conditions, where sailors speed for hours, miles offshore. Any of us could hop off our board anywhere in the bay, stand in chest-deep water to relax or schmooze, surrounded by high-rises on the island, the distant mainland, the Queen Isabella Causeway connecting the two, and the unending bay to the north, over which the best winds come as occasional "northers."*

My eighty-four-year-old father had called me a week prior to advise me that he was checking himself into the hospital the next day. He was to undergo testing for pacemaker eligibility. Although he had repeatedly and forcefully stated "no more hospitals," he indicated no alarm, leading me to believe that he felt the testing was a small thing.

We surmised that his newfound resolve to move back to Colorado near both of his children gave him renewed purpose and tempered his resistance to being in the hospital again. It quickly became apparent that my father was wrong in his risk assessment.

Mort, ever independent, had labored with his walker, lowered himself onto his motorized scooter, and sped away from his newly built, splendidly decorated assisted living apartment, through the halls and down to his car. He loaded the scooter into the back of the Silhouette van using its electric winch, drove himself to the medical center, and had himself admitted.

Several days later, my sister Judy got wind that things had changed. She flew down to assist. After several days there, her resources severely taxed, she called and asked me to come immediately.

I hastily arranged to stow my car stuffed with sailing gear on the island. The next morning I flew to south Florida, rented a car, and arrived at my dad's hospital room at about 7:30 p.m.—whereupon, after a brief greeting, his first words were to call a meeting to order and begin declaring his intentions.

FOR THOSE IN ACUTE NEED OR CRISIS

IF ANY ONE OF US HAS NOT executed a suite of Power Documents, or if the documents are not readily available to present to entities at a moment's notice, we are at a very serious disadvantage.

WITHOUT A SUITE OF POWER DOCUMENTS, WE WILL POTENTIALLY CEDE CONTROL OVER OUR PERSONAL MEDICAL AND FINANCIAL DESTINY TO STRANGERS AND THE COURTS. Should a serious conflict develop between any involved parties, personal representatives may have to work, or even fight, to legally gain and exert control -- with no guarantee of success. Your loved one will languish should such a conflict ensue.

THERE IS NO SUBSTITUTE FOR HAVING AND USING THESE LEGAL INSTRUMENTS. IF POSSIBLE, DROP EVERYTHING AND GET THEM -- NOW.

At the least, you can get the forms for free. Forms are available online. Do two searches with a search engine: one for "YourStateName advance directive" (example: Colorado advance directive) and a second for "YourStateName power of attorney." The first will yield links for Living Wills and Medical Power of Attorney. The second will yield links for Financial Power of Attorney.

Additionally, a Living Will form may be available from the hospital administration office. You'll also want a separate HIPAA Authorization and Release. These are the MINIMUM three documents you need to direct your loved one's treatment.

Whether or not document signatures must be witnessed and who can serve as witnesses may vary from state to state.

HOWEVER, even the basic documents have their legal complexities. While it's better to have self-drafted documents instead of none at all, there is no substitute for competent legal advice and guidance. For the most secure and up-to-date coverage potential, have a law firm prepare the documents. The law firm should be at least moderately sized so that the odds will be better that a lawyer or paralegal will be available to help you immediately should a need arise.

Power Documents: The Only Way to Make Effective and Binding Declarations

MANAGING A SERIOUS HOSPITALIZATION (is there any other kind?) begins long before it occurs, perhaps while we are in perfect health, including full mental faculties. It begins with soul searching and open discussions with family members or other loved ones regarding your healthcare directives and making effective legal declarations that ensure your wishes will be met. Putting declarations into enforceable form results in a set of legal documents I call Power Documents. Without these, your patient-family may literally have no power over your affairs. In a worst-case scenario, doctors and hospitals could proceed entirely on the basis of their values, not yours—even to the extent of excluding a spouse from medical information and decision-making.

At least seven documents comprise a complete documentation set. Five comprise what I call the Power Documents—the ones that ensure control over healthcare matters. Control over everything that is vital in your family's worldly future depends on the contents of the power document set (plus a last will and testament and family trust).

Admitting to any medical institution without having effective Power Documents is flirting with disaster. Undergoing any surgical procedure without having effective Power Documents is inviting it. The documents are:

- The Medical Durable Power of Attorney
- The HIPAA[30] Authorization and Release
- The Living Will
- The Financial Durable Power of Attorney
- The Do Not Resuscitate (DNR) form.

What Happens With and Without the Power Documents?

None of these legal documents is required by any entity. They exist to protect our personal rights and control over our fate. When these documents exist and are presented in a timely manner, doctors and financiers become obligated to do what we want and refrain from doing what we don't want.

However, the treatment group may present limitations, so you, as your loved one's personal representative, will need to have one or more heart-to-heart conversations with each individual in the treatment group to present patient-family wishes and discover if any treatment group member has a problem or conflict in abiding by them.

In the absence of Power Documents, hospitals and doctors may make an effort to identify the patient's closest relative or friend and try to ascertain the patient's wishes. But they are not obligated to constrain their treatment. To the contrary. When the medical documents don't exist or aren't presented, the medical team will provide the treatment it sees fit on the schedule it sees fit, to the extent it sees fit, according to a system that values keeping people alive in any form and at all costs until even the most vigorous mechanical intervention fails. They may perceive potential liability if they do anything other than apply every medical intervention known against dying.

When the Financial Durable Power of Attorney doesn't exist, you cannot obtain or manage funds from your loved one's accounts.

Do I Need a Lawyer to Prepare These Documents?

While these documents are available from multiple sources online, if you can afford a lawyer, it's a good idea to engage one. Lawyers are attuned to the changing legal climate and whatever new clauses may be advisable to include in a document. For example, several attorneys brought to my attention various methods of protecting family access to HIPAA-protected medical records. One loophole was closed by a clause in the lawyer's form that I hadn't seen in online forms; executing a totally separate HIPAA release form outside of the medical POA closed another loophole.

Some lawyers may charge relatively small fees for the powers of attorney and HIPAA release, and very modest fees for a will and trust (in the $25 and $250 ranges per document, respectively). If on a tight budget, do not necessarily write legal assistance off for these invaluable legal tools. Call around for rates, and you might be pleasantly surprised.

Are These Documents Universally Accepted?

Power Documents executed in one state ought to be accepted in all other states. If you have changed residence, however, it's best to execute new ones that are written in and for the new state of residence and to research state statutes that control the circumstances these documents address. If consulting with a lawyer, use one within your residence jurisdiction.

What is a Power of Attorney?

A Power of Attorney is a document. The document names one or more persons known as *proxies* or *agents*. Colloquially, people seem to use and understand POA, as in "I am my father's medical POA." POA is also an abbreviation for the document itself. I use POA to refer to both the documents and the agents throughout this book, as we do in every-day conversation.

When do Powers of Attorney Take Effect?

Some people want these documents to become effective when they sign them (remember that a proxy can only take *control* when the signer becomes incapacitated—this is the most typical scenario). Alternatively, we can specify other times and conditions that must be met before a representative becomes legally empowered to represent us.

Durability

"Durable" in legalise means that the powers granted by the document remain in effect. This is critically important for obvious reasons— if the Power of Attorney "sunsets", that is, ends at some point in time because durability was not written into it, which person or entity will end up in control? To prevent any ambiguity or loss of control, consider executing Durable Medical and Financial Power of Attorney documents. Remember, the powers granted by these documents can be changed at any time simply by executing new ones that include a stipulation saying that they supersede any previously signed POAs.

Single or Multiple Personal Representatives

One or several persons might be named as medical or financial POAs. When more than one person is named, the maker might specify that they must make decisions jointly or, if one is unavailable or unable to act, that the other can make decisions unilaterally.

Power of Attorney Documents Go Stale Over Time

This vital point is rarely broadcast: Institutions may be less likely to accept power of attorney documents that are more than one year old, and they might well reject documents any older.

An aging Financial Power of Attorney is like an old check. Banks won't cash checks over six months old, let alone years old. Financiers in general may unilaterally choose not to honor financial POAs older than one year. Medical system representatives may prefer to see a Medical Power of Attorney that has been signed within the past year, but in general will accept much older ones. I don't know why the financial and medical worlds differ in this regard. Regardless, it means that everyone executing a Financial Power of Attorney must either re-execute the entire document annually or refresh its signature page annually. Put this task on your calendar for every new year.[31] The cost should be minimal to nothing.

If you want to double check what hospitals in your area accept, call their risk management offices and inquire. At this writing, my lawyer counseled me to re-execute the signatory page of my Financial Power of Attorney annually. Professional participants at an end-of-life panel discussion suggested doing the same for the Medical Power of Attorney. My sister's lawyer had her sign a separate single-page form that refers to her POA documents, restating that they represent her directives and remain in effect. As with all legal matters, for the best odds of coverage without loopholes, seek legal advice in the jurisdiction in which you live.

The Medical Durable Power of Attorney Document

THE MEDICAL DURABLE POWER OF ATTORNEY grants one or more persons the authority to make medical decisions for the signer if s/he becomes incapacitated and unable to make decisions. The medical POA speaks directly for the incapacitated patient, issuing treatment directives to medical providers.

Specify Who has Access to the Medical Records

The Health Insurance Portability and Accountability Act (HIPAA) combined with the move toward electronic health records has raised institutional resolve to guard patient healthcare information. This includes your loved one's hospital record (chart), even as it evolves during their treatment, regardless of whether or not you've been told of your loved one's condition by the treatment group.

If you are your loved one's POA, make sure that the Medical Power of Attorney document includes a statement granting you complete and total access to all of your loved one's medical records with no exceptions or preconditions. Restrictions on this vital information have become extreme, excluding even spouses from reviewing their loved one's records and chart in the absence of explicit instructions allowing them access (and regardless of how deeply they may be engaged in caring for their hospitalized loved one).[32]

In this regard, a relatively new document has emerged as a key element of one's Power Docs suite, addressing HIPAA requirements directly.

The HIPAA Authorization and Release Document

THE HIPAA AUTHORIZATION AND RELEASE is a crucial document that directs medical providers to release private health information to the person(s) named. Your reach as personal representative can be severely limited if access to HIPAA-protected medical information is not expressly directed, independent of any other document or patient condition.

This release comes into play in two circumstances. First, in the event that you want to name someone to have access to your medical records but do not want to name that person as your medical POA.

Next, it can guarantee release of medical records in the event of a treatment group versus patient-family dispute over what constitutes incapacitation. Imagine the following conundrum: the Medical POA authorization depends upon the principal being decreed as incapacitated. If a dispute were to develop over that status, the family would require their loved one's medical records to attempt to prove incapacitation. Without the stand-alone HIPAA release, the treatment group would be required to adhere only to the medical POA document. That POA might authorize release of HIPAA-protected medical records only after the patient is decreed incapacitated. Until that time, the records would not be released. If the treatment group refused to recognize and designate the patient as incapacitated, the POA would have to go to court to seek an injunction against them. Meanwhile, your loved one languishes and the bills mount.

The circular dependency described above may sound far-fetched. Good lawyers alert us to potential hazards and how to protect ourselves against them. In these matters especially, it pays to listen closely to their guidance.

The Living Will (Advance Directive) Document

LIVING WILLS ENUMERATE A RANGE OF CONDITIONS and our desired treatment (or lack of treatment) should they arise. This document is *the* primary guide for personal representatives, who will base their decisions on its contents. The Living Will also informs providers of our wishes, which they'll want to know in order to feel most comfortable when dealing with a personal representative.

A Living Will provides life-and-death instructions, and the more specifically desires are stated, the easier a representative's task will be.

In the event that various family members attempt to enforce differing outcomes for a critically ill patient, the Living Will can serve to minimize or eliminate debate as to what ought to occur.

Living Wills come as ready-made forms. They are available online (search for "Living Will" or "advance directive" plus your state name). Lawyers and hospitals have them, too. One interesting alternative to the pro-forma Living Will is the more casually written "Five Wishes." As of this writing, this document, available at www.AgingWithDignity.org, can be purchased for $5 and freely copied. It's a multi-page document with a comparatively manicured look and feel. It is accepted in most, but not all, states. There's value in using it to collect your thoughts, although the lawyers I've spoken with prefer either state-specific boilerplate documents or to create their own customized documents.

Note that a Living Will is a totally different document from a Last Will and Testament, and it serves a different purpose.

Adding Living Will Content to the Medical Power of Attorney

Some attorneys advise against Living Wills on the grounds that doctors don't like them, presumably because they are not an ironclad legal document like a power of attorney. His suggestion is to add all the instructions that typically appear in a Living Will to the Medical Power of Attorney document. Check with your own lawyer about this option.

Pondering Living Will Issues

I suspect that when most families discuss Living Will issues, the unspoken scenarios that we have in mind seem to be black-and-white in nature: the proverbial car wreck or "getting run over by a bus," where one ends up with lost limbs, paralyzed from the neck down, or in a vegetative state, with many years left to live in a highly compromised condition.

I've learned through experience that Living Will issues may play out differently than we imagined when discussing them around the dining room table. In both my parents' cases, their circumstances were not quite as clear-cut. My mother had trouble breathing and quickly wound up unconscious and intubated on a ventilator. My father wound up with multiple infections, debilitated, and in severe pain, with choice points that took almost three weeks to sequentially appear.

Although my mother's medical "crash"[33] was for practical purposes instant with immediate and dramatic effect, we didn't know whether or not it was reversible. We adult children felt within the first week that it was not. Dad, however, was reluctant to let go.

My father crashed in a slightly softer way. Although his condition rather quickly changed from fully functional (if compromised) to debilitated, some weeks passed before we ascertained that his life was indeed threatened.

As our father's medical representatives during what turned out to be Dad's terminal hospitalization, my sister and I learned through simple experience that the directive my father authored (including the document itself, our dining room conversations, and his periodic, consistent proclamations against further hospitalization) were at odds with the fact that he was in the hospital in the condition he was in. The result was that we were at a loss for the clear guidance we thought we had through the document and proclamations. In other words, you can write and proclaim all you want, but if you select hospitalization, the way your demise plays out will be subject to the values of curative medicine and the nature of hospital institutions (which are fraught with all the problems introduced earlier and dissected throughout this book).

Specifying our desires requires that we discover and state our viewpoints regarding what a meaningful life consists of. The challenge is that this may change as we age. We cannot fully know how we'll feel when actually reaching advanced age or a life-threatening medical crisis, whichever comes first. It's all conjecture.

The idea is to offer specific guidance to a personal representative so that s/he has little or nothing to assume about your wishes. Conjecturing takes time, which can evaporate during medical emergencies, and can be emotionally traumatizing anytime, especially when life hangs in the balance.

The guidance continuum ranges from directing that life support continue forever (one's body can be sustained for decades on machines, and special facilities exist that are dedicated to housing what remains of persons in this condition) to mandates never to be hospitalized. The latter may be very hard to adhere to, especially in an emergency "on the street" and if one is not elderly.

Revisit the Living Will periodically to see if it still reflects your values, ethics, outlook, and—most importantly—the lessons of experience. After revising or refreshing a stale Living Will, best practice is to reclaim and shred any old copies. Be sure to redistribute copies of the new document.

Remember that careful attention to a Living Will may save not only us from a destiny we would rather avoid, but will also save personal representatives the angst of making life-and-death decisions in the absence of knowing our wishes.

Living wills do not replace the Medical Power of Attorney. Nor does a Living Will replace a personal representative who knows your wishes. Ideally, the representative knows what you want—not through the Living Will document retrieved from your freezer or safe deposit box and read hurriedly at your hospital bedside, but through deep relationship and open conversations with you.

The Do Not Resuscitate (DNR) Form

RESUSCITATION IS THE MEDICAL ACT OF ATTEMPTING TO REVIVE a body by restarting the heart or lungs after one or both have stopped.

A person for whom breathing or heartbeat has stopped has biologically died.[34] Resuscitation is no caress; it's a seriously invasive set of procedures that have about a five percent chance of success. (See "The Complete Do-Not-Resuscitate Conversation," Chapter 7, for a comprehensive discussion about resuscitation.)

Do not resuscitate (DNR) forms differ by state and must be signed by a physician to be effective. DNRs typically apply to people in grave medical condition, such as the elderly or those with advanced terminal disease.

DNRs are used for patients who are bedded in medical institutions. When not in a medical institution, anyone not wanting resuscitation would execute a no-CPR (cardiopulmonary resuscitation) directive. This also requires a physician's signature to take effect. The signed directive can be supplemented by a bracelet or medallion. After the doctor has signed off on DNR eligibility, the DNR medallion or bracelet may be obtained from your state government. Presumably, first responders would see this object and refrain from resuscitation efforts. DNR status must be shown to emergency responders or they *will* commence resuscitation. After first responders have begun resuscitation, they can stop only if their prolonged and escalating efforts fail or upon a doctor's direct order.

Resuscitation is not a simple issue; many of its aspects and ramifications are left unspoken by the medical profession. "The Complete Do-Not-Resuscitate Conversation" is devoted to exploring what the medical establishment, in my experience, hides from public view regarding resuscitation complexities.

The Financial Durable Power of Attorney Document

THE FINANCIAL DURABLE POWER OF ATTORNEY gives one or several persons the right and authority to engage in transactions on behalf of the person (the *principal*) who executes the document.

When the Financial Power of Attorney Ends

A critical aspect of the Financial Power of Attorney is that the principal must be alive (and most likely incapacitated) in order for the named proxy to transact on their accounts. However, once the principal dies, their Financial Power of Attorney ceases to have any effect—there's no longer a person to represent! This is not relevant for heath matters, but is most definitely an issue for financial matters (and could become relevant medically if funds are needed to pay for certain treatments).

Other Legal Documents: Wills and Trusts

WILLS AND TRUSTS ARE BEYOND THE SCOPE OF THIS BOOK,[35] but they deserve mention because they, too, are critical Power Documents. The aforementioned Power Documents address medical issues; wills and trusts address financial, inheritance, and estate issues.

Unless you want the state to take about twenty-five percent of an estate's value[36] and add six to twelve months to the time it takes for survivors to receive its proceeds, ensure that a will is made. Trusts can be simple or complex and depend completely upon family circumstances and goals. The simplest trust—affording protection for uncomplicated family situations—can be embedded in a will. Some lawyers say that every family, even if made up of only two people, should have a trust. It keeps things, well, in the family.

These two documents ensure that estate assets can be quickly and directly transferred from the estate to the survivors. Just do them.

What Makes Power Documents Effective?

ESSENTIALLY, WHAT MAKES DOCUMENTS EFFECTIVE is that those to whom we present them assess them as valid, and therefore will do what we say. These documents do not take effect because they are signed and sitting in a file at home—they must be shown.

Because the issues these documents cover are considered by many to be the most vital, they require legally acceptable writing and signing.

Validity and effectiveness require that these documents:
- Grant the right powers
- Designate primary and secondary personal representatives
- Are signed and witnessed by the right number and the right people in the right setting with the right credentials
- Are accessible to you when you need them

- Are acceptable to those to whom you present them
- Are recorded by those to whom you present them
- Remain current and don't go "stale."

Grant the Right Powers

Only lawyers can advise you about the contents of medical and financial powers of attorney. It seems to me that legal concepts that used to be sufficiently expressed in few statements now require multiple statements intended to close every imaginable loophole and cover all contingencies. The point is, even if the directive is basic ("I authorize my son Moe to make all decisions and authorize all actions with regards to all my finances and all my property."), a Durable Power of Attorney document states this redundantly in many ways that evidently serve to protect, from various angles, against potential legal or bureaucratic challenges. Contact a lawyer to learn how frequently the legal boilerplate for these documents changes in your state.

Designate Primary and Secondary Representatives

Consider the importance of designating an alternative representative in case the primary representative is unwilling or unable to serve. Remember, without legally-binding personal representation, medical practitioners, institutions, and even governmental agency personnel may end up making critical decisions better left to individuals.

Correct Signing and Witnessing

Signing requirements vary based on the document and the state in which the principal executing it resides. In general, the initial signing usually occurs at a law office, witnessed by at least two unrelated people who will also sign. One of the witnesses must also be a registered notary and will stamp and/or emboss each document. Witnesses sign the last page of a multi-page document, and the principal must initial every document page in addition to signing at the end. Initialization, signing, an adequate number of witnesses, plus notarization is the gold standard of validation.

Accessible Documentation

The Power Documents will do neither you nor your loved one any good if they are unavailable when they're needed.

Assuming a loved one is near-terminal and does not want resuscitation, the most critical document to have on their refrigerator or person is the DNR form (or bracelet). When first responders are called (whether on the street or in the hospital, and even if they are called in error), they will arrive quickly, act immediately, and are virtually impossible to call off (they are under legal constraints).

The next most critical document is the Medical Power of Attorney. If your loved one can't speak for himself, you must be able to speak in his place. If challenged as to your authority to do so, only the document, and not your assertion, will prove that you are authorized.

The Living Will and Financial Power of Attorney documents also need to be accessible. While immediate accessibility is best, depending upon your situation, it may be that next-day access will work OK.

Acceptable Documentation

I was never asked for an original power document; copies always sufficed. This is not to say that an original would never be required. After dealing with the requirements of various entities during estate settlement, my suggestion is to be prepared for anything. Original or copy, you have to have the document in question or go get it; if an entity requires proof, it won't take your word for anything. This implies several things:

- Multiple copies of each set of such documents need to be safely stored in several locations. Locations include at the draftee's home, a safe deposit box, the lawyer's office, and the home and safe deposit box of each personal representative.
- You must remember to take these documents with you at the onset of a medical emergency, especially if it is out of town or state.

During my father's hospitalization, my sister, who arrived on the scene before me, was queried to authenticate her POA status. Otherwise, his doctors seemed to recognize and authenticate responsible family members (me), perhaps by virtue of my having shown up (few other people showed up and none stayed on a regular basis) and trusting that I was, indeed, the brother and son. I had so much to attend to that I didn't think to ask the providers why they didn't request to see my Power Documents and/or proof of identity.

During my research, one doctor mentioned to me that when families exhibit contentiousness among themselves, the physicians get more attentive to who in the family is the designated Medical Power of Attorney. Due to what we considered adequate advance planning within an open, communicative family with shared values, my family was of like mind as we helped my father manage his dying process. Perhaps our congruence was apparent and that was why we weren't challenged more rigorously.

When in Doubt

If you are not using a lawyer to prepare your Power Documents, take care to understand and verify that they will work. Research your state government websites online and question several hospitals about which publicly available forms they will accept.

The Size of the Law Firm and Power Documents

ANY COMPETENT LAWYER CAN ADVISE YOU on Power Documents and prepare a suite for you. There is one area, however, where a firm with several attorneys and their support personnel can offer you better service than a solo law practice and its secretary and paralegal.

That area is urgent support. Should problems arise for which you'd need legal advice or legal representation on short notice, a larger firm will be more likely to be able to provide it. Solo law practices, although corporations, may function more like sole proprietorships. A lawyer may be tied up in court for days at a time. If that lawyer is the only one in the firm, you might be waiting those days for his attention—days which you may not have if you need legal assistance for medical matters or if you want to transact certain estate assets before returning to your home half a continent from your deceased loved one.

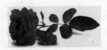

Power Documents Recap: What You Can Do

If your loved one is hospitalized, document everything throughout each day and night. Maintain notes (your personal "chart") or keep a journal.

Be an effective question-asker! *Start now.* Has this chapter answered all your questions about:

- Which legal documents are vitally important and what they enable?
- Whether any of these documents are required?
- How to prepare these documents?
- Where the documents are accepted?
- What happens when these documents exist?
- What happens when these documents do not exist?
- What to ponder when creating these documents?
- How often to update these documents?
- What makes the documents effective?

If you do not have all the information you need, write your questions down. How will you get them answered? Reread this chapter? Internet research? Library research? Consulting with family and friends? A phone call to a professional or organization? Go online or pick up the phone book, find a likely contact, and send the email or place the call.

SECTION 2 | EFFECTIVELY MANAGE HOSPITALIZATION

THE HOSPITALIZATION SECTION examines a range of incidents that typically occur in hospitals. Some may be known to you; many are probably not. If you haven't experienced them for yourself, you won't know about them, because hospitals don't tell you.

I will point out, clearly and uncompromisingly, hospital faults as my family experienced them. I'll untangle what leads to grave conditions with grievous consequences, some of which I consider malpractice (as in "bad professional practices," distinct from bad medicine, although the lines do blur). I'll state my conclusions in direct terms.

By the end of this section, you'll know how to avoid experiences similar to ours as much as is possible. You'll also understand my family's felt responses to our experiences and why you should avoid our fate. Although I stated this in the preface, it bears repeating: *My goal is that you understand both intellectually and emotionally the conditions and events a family is likely to endure when dealing with end-of-life hospitalizations in the hope that you will act to preclude unnecessary pain.*

It would be easy to sidestep criticizing these institutions because they, and treatment providers who work in them, improve and save lives. Sidestepping would be wrong, because their way of serving induces angst among their patient-families. It would be doubly wrong, because for those facing end of life, the conditions I'll describe infringe on precious, irreplaceable moments in the days prior to death.

In critiquing hospitals, it's important to differentiate between the services they provide. These include emergency trauma care (the emergency room in the Emergency Department, or ED), walk-in specialty clinics, short-term stays for acute problems (like broken bones and non-catastrophic surgeries), and finally, the area this book focuses on: extended hospitalizations of a week or more, typically near or at the end of life.

Because of the many personal circumstances resulting in hospitalization, it may help readers to approach this section with some mental flexibility. Much of what I present here is applicable to almost any hospitalization. Because any hospitalization can shift from serious to *very* serious, one might say this presentation can apply to every hospitalization. And because this book emanates from my family's particularly egregious felt responses during two terminal hospitalizations, my recurring focus includes profound issues arising during end of life and the weeks leading to it.

This conversation focuses primarily on the ways hospitals function and how this impacts patient-families. In this respect, the healthcare industry is like the stereotypical "geek," a technically skilled person who's uncomfortable with everyday social discourse. That's of little consequence at a dinner party, and of enormous consequence when your loved one is dying in a geek-like environment—especially when the institutions proclaim far and wide that they provide loving care (which is, plainly, false advertising).

Hospitals differ from one another in many ways. These include policies, staffing, hierarchy, culture, and more. Use the information in this section as a guide. Ask, ask, ask, to clarify how things work at any institution your loved one is bedded within.

Chapter 3, "Differing Sensibilities: Care and Communication in Hospitals," analyzes the schism we experience due to the related issues of what constitutes care and the communication disconnect between the medical establishment and laypersons. We will reorient our thinking about what hospitals are and provide (and to who), so as no longer to be blinded by what we wish them to be and to do. We'll acquire a list of the things we most need to learn about hospitals in order to function effectively within them.

Chapter 4, "Family Involvement in Hospital Care," briefly overviews working conditions inside hospitals and presents a range of typical problems, focusing primarily on the treatment and role of the family half of the patient-family.

Chapter 5, "Forecasting and Ethical Support: What You Need to Know, When You Need to Know It, and How to Get It," introduces the important, overarching issues of obtaining timely, relevant, and substantive information from providers during the entirely of your hospitalization, and how to use hospital resources to help you obtain practical and ethical guidance.

Chapter 6, "Who's Where, When, Why, for How Long and Other Turns through the Hospital Maze," presents another range of practical issues to help you effectively manage your loved one's hospitalization, this time focusing primarily on the various treatment group members who come and go and what to do in relation to them under various circumstances.

Chapter 7, "The Complete Do-Not-Resuscitate Conversation," presents a one-of-a-kind, in-depth look at the many issues comprising resuscitation—a circumstance with profound implications that shadows every hospitalization, yet is not ever, as far as I know, comprehensively explained to the hospital-going public.

3 | Differing Sensibilities: Care and Communication in Hospitals

M
Y EIGHTY-YEAR-OLD MOTHER, RUTH, had developed periodic cardiac arrhythmia (irregular heartbeat). She had gone for a cardioversion, a procedure to restore normal heart rhythm. That day her heartbeat was normal; as she waited under observation, she suddenly couldn't breathe. The staff asked her if she wanted breathing assistance. She accepted and was intubated (a breathing tube was inserted into her trachea). As far as I know, she went from there to unconsciousness in the critical care unit of a local hospital.

In a heroic scheduling feat, within some hours of Dad's mid-morning call, my sister Judy and I rendezvoused to board a four-hour non-stop flight, arriving at our parent's home in a rental car at one o'clock in the morning.

Several hours later, in the critical care unit, we found my mother with a very low internal temperature (94°F) under a single, thin top sheet. I was told (several days later) that she was the most critically ill patient in the entire facility. We were shocked to learn how little had been done to elevate her body temperature—not even as much as would occur in a youngster's bedroom.

I want to suggest that you keep a fleece blanket in the trunk of your car and bring it up to the hospital room if it's needed, because it seems ridiculous and even life-threatening to wait for something as basic as shelter to be offered a freezing patient in critical care. I want to suggest this, but I can't. It's not feasible. Don't do it. If you bring the thing into intensive care, you have a real breach of hygiene due to dirt and germs it may contain. But without adequate covering over your loved one, you may stand around while s/he shivers, waiting for the system to provide basic warmth (almost two days in my mother's case). Your options? Harangue the staff to get some covering on their patient, or throw your own coat over him or her (and see if this gets you thrown out of the unit). Either one may earn you the designation of a "problem family."

FOR THOSE IN ACUTE NEED OR CRISIS

HOSPITALS PROVIDE BODILY REPAIR SERVICES, not care as you and I understand the term. Doctors provide treatment. Nurses provide periodic monitoring. YOU AND YOUR LOVED ONE'S FAMILY MUST PROVIDE THE CARE. This may be confusing when you experience it -- all the more so because you are not told that this is generally how the system works.

WE ARE NOT NAIVE. There's a communication schism. Hospitals and lay people like you and I define the word "care" differently.

Hospitals communicate to us through banners, lobby placards, brochures, advertisements, website images, and posters. These items tell us things the hospital wants us to hear, but contain almost nothing we really need to know (with the exception of legally binding patient rights statements).

What we really need to know are a host of things aside from how wonderful the hospital we're in is in their opinion. WE NEED TO KNOW VITAL THINGS such as:

• How our loved one's doctors function, alone and together, and when they'll be around so we can be there to hear their assessments directly.

• How the hospital functions, and how our loved one's treatment will proceed, so we will understand why we wait.

• The kinds of DECISIONS THAT MAY BE LOOMING, so we can discuss them and come to emotional terms with them in case we need to make them. We need to know this in advance so we're not taken by surprise (shocked).

• The range of medical people who will be attending to our loved one, how to tell them apart from one another, and the range of treatment services each is licensed to provide.

• What to do if and when a medical provider, from technician to doctor, makes mistakes or mistreats our loved one.

• HOW TO FIND ASSISTANCE, in and from the hospital, if we find ourselves not knowing how, or feeling unable, to make a decision about our loved one's treatment, or if we and a provider disagree on our loved one's treatment.

The Significance of Communication and the Shock of its Absence

AS WE AWAITED ADEQUATE COVERINGS FOR MY MOTHER, we were all frozen in her ICU room. She was cold due to her depressed internal and skin temperatures, and the family was frozen in bewilderment. It's a foreboding environment, absent the loving care we expect.

Having reflected upon two parent's end-of-life hospitalizations that unfolded over a total of approximately six weeks' time, I conclude that medical practitioners and the rest of us are not speaking the same language. We have different understandings of what constitutes "care."

Hospitals are responsible for this schism. Care in the healthcare context is something virtually every one of us has experience with, either as a recipient of care from a loved one or as a caregiver to a loved one at home. Hospitals imply strongly that their performance as caregivers is the same. It's not, and they never tell us what their definition of care is.

Hospitals have not communicated with us about what they actually provide. More precisely, they seem to communicate only what they want us to think, not what families need to know once a loved one is bedded in their institution. Although individual treatment providers are part of the problem, the root cause is institutional.

Although for most of us care and communication are inseparable, in the hospital setting they are not. Organizationally, care and communication occupy different territory in the hospital landscape. Communication is undertaken by administration. Caregivers provide care. However, in the patient-family experience, care and communication are inseparable, as tightly entwined as the snake around the staff of Asclepius, the ancient and modern medical symbol.[37]

The way lay people approach hospitalization and what we expect there emanates from our experiences in our own bedrooms. We have a common understanding about what care consists of. When our expectations for care go unmet at the hospital bedside, we experience a disconnect at best and shock at worst. When commonly understood parameters of care continue to go unmet throughout a hospitalization, our shock continues and creates disorientation. Repetitive shock adds up to a disturbing cumulative experience that interferes with patient-family functioning and decision-making.

The result, during serious-to-terminal hospitalization, is systemic disorientation of the patient-family. The only solution to disorientation is education—clear, helpful guidance by the system about how it functions and how we must function within it. Without such communication, at those times, we feel that the care our loved one deserves is inexplicably compromised.

In this chapter I suggest that without comprehensive, well-delivered communication from both hospitals and providers, care is compromised. It is incomplete. Without communication we are adrift, unable to adequately assess our surroundings, our role, and our loved one's future.

A holistic understanding of how communication forms an intrinsic part of care will occur in a heartbeat. It came about for me upon realizing that although my parents were the patients, we family members were simultaneously an unacknowledged part of the treatment group. As such we were entitled to some purposeful attention and assistance, if not care, from the hospitals and providers in order to fulfill our role as personal representatives—a role largely unacknowledged by the system.

Earlier, we discussed how to *be* a personal representative. We have not yet examined the circumstances that arise that require us to accompany our loved ones throughout their hospitalization, let alone become actively involved. That examination begins by untangling the confusion around care and communication offered by hospitals to their customers.

Redefining Hospitals

BECAUSE OF THE CONFUSION, it's worth restating what hospitals provide:

> **In the context of hospitalization for a serious illness, hospitals do not provide healthcare. In this context, hospitals provide bodily repair services under the direction of independent physician-scientists.**

In the context of serious illness—a protracted hospitalization requiring continuous supervision—hospitals are places of repair, not care or healing. Their operation is geared toward support of physician-scientists, practitioners of bodily repair, the majority of whom are independent of the hospital. Hospital treatment is actually the application of science and technology to attempt to inhibit, reverse, or cure bodily ailments.

Before an ailment can be treated, it must be diagnosed. Treatment is then applied to the ailment. The ailment takes center stage; the person who is the subject of the disease and the people around that person (you and your family) are considered peripheral to the proceedings.

In contrast, healing is a human process that, at its most effective, includes the biomechanics and chemistry of repair plus attendance to the patient after and between medical interventions. Caring is a human endeavor, providing nurture and support, oriented toward ongoing physical, emotional, and spiritual needs. In our experience, hospitals do not provide this type of care for their patient-family customers.

Nor do hospital operations support families, unless you know how to find the people or programs whose function is to do this and to enroll their help. (Determining if family support structures exist at an institution and how to recruit and leverage them is the topic of the forecasting chapter). In any case, expect to actively seek and stimulate (pester) staff to give you the information you deserve, need, and are entitled to.

All this is despite what one clinical ethicist described to me as hospitals' primary mission: providing nursing care. Paraphrasing our conversation, she suggested that since many surgeries now occur on an outpatient basis, the primary remaining function of hospitals is to nurse their seriously ill patients back to health.[38] Yet hospitals have decimated their nursing staffs in various ways (which I'll present further below), making true nursing care an unattainable goal.

Understanding the distinction between our notion of care and the medical establishment's appropriation of the word care *takes us a long way toward becoming effective personal representatives, because we function with a changed worldview.* By recognizing the difference between our understanding of care and the idiosyncratic use of the term "care" in the healthcare field, we can better know what to expect—and most importantly what *not* to expect—from hospitals and those who provide services there.

Regarding hospitalizations that span weeks, especially for the aged with multiple life-threatening afflictions, the system presents a generally common character to patient-families. Long-term hospitalization, according to my family's experiences, is characterized by:

- An absence of communication with the family
- Systemic indifference to, and disregard for, family needs
- Fragmented treatment management and treatment delivery
- A lack (a total lack, in our two experiences) of meaningful and timely guidance (forecasting)
- Being ignored for extended periods
- In the worst cases, severely limited visitation and patient contact restrictions
- Recurring breaches of hygiene
- The potential for contraction of hospital-borne infection (realized in both of our parents' hospitalizations)
- Inadequate care and/or monitoring
- Denial of inadequate patient and family care by nursing management.

I am not including here the already well-documented instances of clinical mistakes such as medication mishaps, surgical mistakes, unnecessary deaths, etc.[39]

It seems that everyone knows someone who has endured a hospitalization they characterize as terrible, either as a patient or a family member. Whether recent or long past, these experiences remain powerfully lodged. Stories told to me were delivered with outrage and pain even years after their occurrence.

This lingering angst has its roots in the very first moments the family encounters their loved one in the hospital. Predictably, those moments are most difficult if they occur in the Emergency Department.

According to both an emergency department doctor and a Catholic hospital's mission director[40] I queried,

- About 10% of the families of patients admitted to the Emergency Department *present*—medical lingo for "show up" or "appear"—as capable of handling the crisis at its outset (by "capable of handling" I mean able to effectively enter into treatment deliberations that result, within a short period of time, in reasoned decisions without the decision paralysis that would lead to the patient languishing).

- About 20% of the families of patients admitted as inpatients for end-of-life conditions present as capable of handling the hospitalization at its outset.
- Eventually, about 50% of the families of patients admitted as inpatients for end-of-life conditions become capable of managing their loved one's hospitalization and death in concert with the treatment group.

Add to the small numbers of capable families the range of cultural, religious, and ethical considerations, and it is evident that every treatment group has its hands full. The unending stream of lay people into hospitals presents very challenging conditions for treatment providers. This mix of patients and families is every hospital's customer base, and providers have no choice but to make the best of what I imagine adds up to a chaotic parade of characters.

While patient-families differ in their characteristics, their underlying medical problems may generally be more or less the same. How about hospitals? Are hospitals more or less the same? Do we stand the same chance for confusion about treatment due to absent, misleading, or poorly delivered communication at every hospital?

How Hospitals Compare

My initial research question was whether it made any substantial difference which hospital a loved one ends up in. Were my family's experiences typical or unique? Is there any meaningful difference between urban and rural hospitals? For-profit or not-for-profit hospitals? Research or community hospitals? Secular or religiously based hospitals? Public or private hospitals?

The consensus among the medical professionals I interviewed was unanimous, confirming my own limited experience. Regarding basic functioning and problems patient-families are susceptible to, the various types of American hospitals are identical. The potential for the difficulties I discuss is universal across hospital types nationwide.

One exception may be religiously based hospitals. Because of an orientation borne of their mission, religiously based hospitals (which typically have names beginning with "Saint") may already have a heightened awareness of the role good communication plays during patient-family hospitalizations. This results from, and results in, a more humane ethic manifesting itself, if only in a limited form. Community hospitals may be similarly advanced if the communities they serve are relatively forward thinking or well-off; that sensibility may tend to filter into community hospitals almost by osmosis, due to the greater community's social fabric.

Significant differences do exist, however, regarding clinical treatment, hospital culture (which impacts family care), staffing ratios, success statistics, etc. Jari Holland Buck's *Hospital Stay Handbook: A Guide to Becoming a Patient Advocate to Your Loved Ones* provides a useful summary of these very important considerations,[41] specifically related to selecting hospitals based on your below-the-surface screening of their organizational attributes and the resources they offer.[42]

Why We Expect Care From Hospitals

WHY DO WE CONTINUE TO EXPECT a complete range of customer service (care) during hospitalization? Are we naive for expecting care for our hospitalized loved one?

The sentence above contains four key words: *expect, care, hospitals,* and *naive.*

A wise friend of mine asserts that having *expectations* is problematic, because when our expectations go unmet, we tend to *react* rather than *respond.* Perhaps the phrase "preconceived notions" might substitute for "expectations." Living without preconceived notions is a superior skill, for without them one may be better positioned to respond to situations from a place of equilibrium, rather than react to situations emotionally.

Although this level of equanimity may be ideal, it can be hard to maintain an even temper when a loved one is in critical condition, considering the totality of experiences we're subject to. It's difficult not to have expectations of caring treatment from providers upon whom your loved one's life depends.

Care is a loaded notion. It is subject to different interpretations, depending upon who defines it—we as individuals or hospitals as businesses.

Hospitals are institutions with a history and a particular role in today's world that is unique from any other time in their, or our, past. The way they function is particularly opaque; hospitals are neither transparent nor forthcoming.

When pondering if we are naive in expecting that hospitals provide care, several questions arise: What do we mean by "care"? Why do we expect it of hospitals?

What you and I mean by "care" is the applied presence of round-the-clock compassionate attendance. Attentiveness. The care we learned at home, primarily from our mothers. It's the care we now provide to our spouses and our own children, and the care we want provided to our family members and elderly parents. I call this *Mom-and-Apple-Pie Care.*

And if we have a preconceived notion that hospitals deliver Mom-and-Apple-Pie Care, it's due to two things: hospitals used to provide it, as recently as the 1960s, and hospitals proactively communicate to us that they continue to provide care today.

What Hospitals Communicate Serves Hospitals, Not Patient-Families

Several things distinguish effective communication from poor communication. They include:

- Whether communication happens at all
- The communication's substance—it's content and emphasis
- The communication's timeliness
- The medium used to communicate
- Whose interests the communication serves.

By and large, the communications that hospitals project toward the public serve the marketing goals of the institution. The communication package does not address the vital needs of patient-families. I find it odd that hospitals misconstrue what constitutes effective communication. After all, a hospital trip is not a vacation. A hospital's reputation does not materialize from the happy images atop clinical white backgrounds in magazine ads, on web pages, or messages displayed on building-sized banners. A hospital's reputation is the direct result of our *experiences* there and how we relate our experiences to family and friends.

We are not naive; Americans understand marketing and advertising for what they are. The problem with healthcare is that the cumulative effect of its marketing communications is not matched by vital instructive information, delivered effectively, throughout each hospitalization. In terms of efficacy, the information and guidance side of the scale is, for practical purposes, entirely empty.

A schism exists. Let's first look at the communications I've encountered at and from hospitals, then we'll examine what we really need to be told by and about hospitals.

Banners as Billboards

One facility we occupied for nearly three weeks hung large banners that were visible from the adjacent roadway and which functioned as billboards. The banners touted that this hospital was one of the nation's hundred best. Hundred best what? Based on what? Best for whom? According to whose assessment? The answers were not stated on the banner-billboards.

Another set of "hundred best" banners hung in the dining room. The small type showed that *Working Mother* magazine had voted this hospital as among the hundred best places to work.

Months later, a visit to the hospital website showed that there were two "hundred best" designations running concurrently, with the undefined one apparently relating to quality of care as defined by safety metrics, measured by a hospital accreditation organization. Given the problems my family experienced during my father's hospitalization there, I had not previously made the connection between our experiences and their assertion of being among the best hospitals in the nation.

And neither would you have made a connection without researching and considering what's behind the "hundred best" advertisements. Making a connection is not what these communications are about. Rather, they are about making feel-good associations.

The hospital's website at that time indicated that the exterior banner referred to a designation by The Joint Commission (formerly known as The Joint Commission on Accreditation of Healthcare Organizations —JCAHO—, commonly pronounced as "Jayco"). Accreditation by TJC is to hospitals as state accreditation is to colleges: a desirable designation with bottom line implications.

According to the ethics officer at a local community hospital, The Joint Commission's "hundred best" recognition is based on a series of quality indicators and benchmarks. By any standard, safety metrics are vitally important. The problem is that hospital accreditation does not include, let alone measure *experiential metrics*, vital treatment (here I'll say *care*) families ought to receive, including communication about what does and doesn't occur in hospitals, and why.

Lobby Placards

Every hospital has two placards hanging in its lobby. One is the institutional *Mission Statement* and the other is a statement of *Patient's Rights*.

The Mission Statement is a statement of purpose, hung there so that you and I feel reassured and have a positive impression of the place. It's usually wonderful to read, and alarmingly out of sync with a significant amount of what goes on within the hospital (by "significant," I mean what matters most to the personal representative and family members throughout the course of a loved one's hospitalization).

The Patient's Rights placard is a legal advisory. Many of the listed rights are vital and important to understand. Some patient rights are clearly stated, but not all. One clarification typically lacking has to do with the distinction between refusing examination or treatment and actually firing the person or institution providing examination or treatment. Refusing treatment in general is one thing; desiring treatment but not from a particular individual working within an institution—or not from the institution itself—is quite another. This second "refusal" falls under the topic of firing nurses, doctors, and hospitals. This patient right is not addressed in the placard, but it does exist. Additionally, you may not see reference to firing the institution and moving to a different hospital altogether, or if you do, it may not be stated very clearly. We had to fire a technician and two nurses (one hospital nurse, one hospice intake nurse) during my father's hospitalization, and had we known better, we might have considered firing my mother's hospital by finding another institution for her and ourselves.

Print Advertisements and Website Images

At least one popular national weekly news magazine publishes an annual healthcare issue, and in their 2005 publication I observed a number of full-page advertisements from medical institutions. There seems to be one key ingredient in these ads: the happy couple. Husband and wife golfing. Father and daughter in a schoolroom with the phrase, "my Dad's [insert malady here] operation," written on the blackboard. The happy couple picture is ubiquitous; even as I write this I see on one hospital website a happy couple as part of a composite image topping the webpage. This young woman joyously dances in the hallway with a man who appears to be a doctor, judging from the unusually square, or at least indeterminate, cut of his sky blue coat, a style and color which infers "clinician." I have no idea if hospital management made this particular associative decision, or if they merely didn't nix the hyperbole.

In any case, the message is this: not only do we restore you to active and happy living, we do it with love. Dancing-in-the-halls love. The kind of love expressed by families. These images are infused with love. They leak love. The message we are intended to get is that hospitals apply loving care.

Brochures and Handbooks

Printed materials may actually contain important information for families of hospitalized loved ones. That's a good thing. The problem is that this information is often tucked away where you don't really notice it. Sometimes there is a lack of differentiation or emphasis; other times the problem is ineffective delivery (certain information is more effectively conveyed in isolation from other information, or verbally from person to person). For instance, finding out about patient or family liaison services and the existence and availability of an ethics committee ranks very high on a list of important things to know. I don't think that listing these essential services in a letter-sized trifold brochure or on a sheet in a three-ring binder is adequate.

Imagine arriving at the bedside of a loved one from halfway across the country, distressed, disoriented, and worried. Don't you need something more than the printed word to convey must-know information?

And not every personal representative even sees printed materials, especially if you arrive at your loved one's bedside some days after your loved one has been admitted.

A Note About Naiveté

When discussing medical matters, it's important to distinguish between naiveté that comes in response to advertising and what we actually expect regarding healthcare. Most of us recognize the former for what it is: image-building. Buffed up images are tolerable if balanced by the delivery of the services that are portrayed.

Healthcare consumers are particularly vulnerable when a loved one is hospitalized, and all the more vulnerable when that hospitalization is critical or terminal. End of life requires straight talk from and between all parties, and the institution housing us is no exception. Hospitals continue to trade on our expectations of loving care while systemically providing bodily repair services and, in my experience, imperfect monitoring. It's not like we'll avoid hospitalization when our bodies require serious repair. When the situation warrants, we're hospital customers. Given this, I find hospitals' emphasis on marketing imagery and their simultaneous de-emphasis of truly useful patient-family communications inexplicable. Because of how vital the omitted information is, I think the withholding crosses over the line into bad practice.

Redefining the Patient

HOSPITALIZATION NEAR OR AT END OF LIFE IS DIFFERENT NOW than at any previous time in history. This is due to:

- The impact of advanced technology, which both extends our active lifespan and alters the pattern of dying (changing it from quick to protracted)
- Ethical complexities around life support and resuscitation
- The fragmented nature of treatment delivered in hospitals
- The prevalence of medical mistakes ranging from breaches of

hygiene and errors with medicines to hospital-borne infections and erroneous surgeries

- A general inability to provide nursing care due to lowered staff-to-patient ratios.

Families will continue to gather around their hospitalized loved ones, to wait and commune. But this is no longer enough. Today we must take a more active role as patient representatives and advocates.

The notion of patient advocacy is a curious one. Why should anyone have to advocate for their loved one in a hospital, where doctors practice medicine in accordance with their oath to "first do no harm"?

The fact is that medical care has become extremely fragmented and complex. Most of us have not kept up with the nature of its complexity. Yes, we are aware that ethical problems arise, and occasionally one of them rises above the fold of the daily paper or is featured on the evening newscasts. But a useful understanding of the nature of ethical conundrums and how they play out in real life during hospitalization requires months or years of research and contemplation.

One thing the medical system does discuss openly is the need for patient advocates, although it doesn't explain *why* advocates are necessary. Reasons will emerge throughout this book's hospitalization section.

At this point, accept this: your loved one is at additional risk—perhaps grave—without your oversight. Although you may feel as though you are providing unpaid help to the hospital through your active in-volvement (you are), it is far better than your loved one staying at higher risk due to your absence. We're not so much giving to the hospital as we are protecting our loved one.

Thus the *patient* is really a unit I call the *patient-family*. As of this writing, many, if not most, hospitals fail to formally recognize or serve this unit.

In order for family members to function effectively as patient representatives, we need support. We need humane places to wait and to work on our loved one's behalf. We need notification of treatment phases and continual appraisal of our loved one's current and likely condition. We need computers, internet access, and printers. We need private conference areas for treatment group conferencing. And we need straight, proactive communication.

These are not concierge services pampering to the over-indulged. If hospitals require families to function as unpaid team members advocating for loved ones bedded within, they ought to provide the resources that support that role.

What We Really Need to Know from Hospitals

ARE BANNERS-AS-BILLBOARDS, print advertisements and website images, patient bill of rights and mission statements, brochures and handouts sufficient to support you in your role as a decision-making personal representative?

They are not. They are of little-to-zero value for people needing to know how to function during a loved one's hospitalization. What we as patients, family members, and personal representatives most need to know includes the following:

- An early review of the patient's advance directive and resuscitation status
- Explanation about when and how these directives are actually brought into effect during the hospitalization and how we can verify that they are in effect
- An explanation of the various aspects of hospital time and how procedures and treatment moves through hospital time
- An explanation of the various staff members who might attend to your loved one; their training, skillsets, and responsibilities; and how to differentiate among them
- The nature and limits of patient care
- The nature and limits of family care
- How the treatment group is organized and how it functions, including who is in charge of the treatment group providing for your loved one for the duration of their hospitalization
- Treatment group contact information and descriptions of their backgrounds and training
- When to expect treatment group conferences and who will attend them
- The kinds of decisions that typically arise at choice points— moments requiring decisions—and during treatment conferences

- Patient-family support personnel and how to contact them
- An explanation of under what conditions the patient-family will receive guidance
- A complete and thorough overview of resuscitation (a most important topic, as we'll discuss below)
- Behavioral and physical symptoms of the onset of death
- Procedures to follow when the patient-family is dissatisfied with treatment rendered (or not rendered) by any individual
- Procedures to follow if the patient-family is dissatisfied with the institution as a whole

In cases where the personal representative arrives on the scene some days after patient admission, all this information ought to be provided in a conference convened especially to inform this person of these vital considerations.

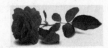

Hospital Care and Communication Recap: What You Can Do

If your loved one is hospitalized, document everything throughout each day and night. Maintain notes (your personal "chart") or keep a journal.

Be an effective question-asker! *Start now.* Has this chapter answered all your questions about:

- Who is the patient during hospitalization?
- Are all hospitals the same, and if not, how do they differ?
- What kind of care do we expect from hospitals?
- Are we naive for expecting it?
- What kind of care do hospitals provide?
- How and what do hospitals communicate?
- What vital things do we really need to be told by hospitals in order to effectively manage our loved one's hospitalization?

If you do not have all the information you need, write your questions down. How will you get them answered? Reread this chapter? Internet research? Library research? Consulting with family and friends? A phone call to a professional or organization? Go online or pick up the phone book, find a likely contact, and send the email or place the call.

4 | Family Involvement in Hospital Care

J UDY ARRIVED AT DAD'S HOSPITAL *about four days after his admission. He was already debilitated from whatever was afflicting him. Being a competent nurse, Judy lifted the lid on his lunch plate to see what he'd eaten only to discoverer that he hadn't eaten at all.*

This was not because he wasn't hungry—to the contrary. It was because he couldn't lift a utensil to his mouth.[43] *Several days prior, he'd ambulated in with a smile on his face; now he was virtually helpless.*

For whatever reasons, neither nurses nor staff members saw to it that Dad got fed. They did not verify his intake and reasons for the lack of it. This, you'd think, would be included as part of basic nursing care in any hospital, let alone in one accredited by The Joint Commission as one of the country's "100 Best."

We hired outside help to come in every day on afternoon and night shifts. Neither Judy nor I could be at the hospital 24/7 (although it's becoming increasingly advocated that a family member remain at the bedside 24/7 to ensure adequate patient care).

We rendezvoused at Dad's bedside each morning at seven o'clock in order to be there when the doctors made their rounds. We stayed through lunchtime and the arrival of the afternoon shift of our hired help. At that time, we returned to our respective bases—Judy to sleep, me to work. Back to the hospital during the dinner hour and the evening, at which point our hired help changed to its second shift, which would last through breakfast, when we'd arrive for the day's first visit and a debriefing. These ladies were there so that Dad would not be alone when we couldn't be there. They were there to spoon-feed him when he was hungry and hold cups with straws for him so that he could drink. They were there because what the nurses provided, partial monitoring according to a schedule, did not provide nor equate to "care."

We spent $200 per day for assistance to ensure that Dad would have help eating and drinking. Given that the hospital charged nearly $90,000 for his two-and-a-half week stay, one might have thought that such basics would have been covered.

FOR THOSE IN ACUTE NEED OR CRISIS

IN TERMS OF PROVIDING CARE (as distinct from treatment), hospitals may have reached their zenith in the mid-twentieth century. Today, the corporate takeover of hospitals coupled with insurance company control over healthcare delivery has changed the healthcare landscape. In particular, fewer nurses attend to more patients, and they are more stressed as they do so. Making matters worse is that patients tend to be sicker, older, and more frail than ever before.

DAILY RISKS TO PATIENTS include germs associated with poor hygiene, hospital-caused infections, and mistakes in administering fluids, IV drips, and medications. You must oversee your loved one's treatment, and must arrange for family-side 24/7 patient coverage. Feel lucky if you are supported in this by the hospital. Do not expect to be comfortable.

Doctors will talk anywhere. Try to carry on discussions in private conference rooms (if any exist and are nearby) rather than public hallways and noisy, crowded waiting rooms.

The admitting physician is supposed to be the medical "team leader." S/he may be so in name but may not be so in fact; it's hard to corral a group of independent specialists. Without a clear and strong team leader, IT'S POSSIBLE THAT NO ONE DOCTOR WILL BE IN CONTROL -- a situation known as "discontinuity of care." Managing discontinuity of care is trying at best, and your loved one may be at more risk as long as it persists.

If at some point you are tempted or need to complain, take it no further than the charge nurse of the wing or unit your loved one occupies. It will be a waste of your time to seek out and engage nursing administration. Beyond the charge nurse, seek in-hospital ethical counselling and support.

Why Hospitals are the Way They Are

HOSPITALS HAVE CHANGED OVER TIME. Those of us middle aged or older have lived through pronounced changes in hospital culture. Understanding those changes can help lessen the extrinsic shock when encountering them.

Aspects that are important to our conversation include:

- How hospitals have changed over time
- How medical technology impacts hospitalization and end of life
- How the corporatization of most hospitals has impacted all hospitals nationally
- The goal of hospital treatment and its relation to health insurance
- The lack of a go-to physician
- What medical anthropology reveals about how end of life is managed by hospitals.

How Hospitals have Changed

For centuries hospitals were truly unhealthy places. Western medicine was in its infancy, and little of what occurred in hospitals was effective.

By the mid-twentieth century, American hospitals had become places where nurses could provide care and, if one was terminal, where one could go to die a peaceful death. This began changing in the 1960s with several changes: artificial life-support technologies, intensive care units, the corporatization of hospitals, and the evolution of our peculiar health insurance system.

For some years (coinciding with your childhood and teen years, if you're a Baby Boomer), hospitals indeed provided Mom-and-Apple-Pie Care. This care was real. We remember it, and it is those now-distant scenes that the ubiquitous "happy couple" marketing tries to resuscitate. Generally, until approximately the 1960s, dying was either quick (the collapse at home or on the job) or people died of old age. If hospitalized, they faded away over days or weeks. There were no ethical conundrums about extending life because few diseases could be rolled back, and there were no life-support alternatives.

The introduction of mechanical and chemical life support coupled with body repairs that extend active lives by decades has created consequences we all live with today. It's no surprise that intensive care units were developed about the same time as the first ventilators and other life-extending machinery. Now when our bodies fail, they fail differently than if the interventions had never been introduced. After years of life-extending interventions, when you finally begin your terminal failure, you're older and frailer than in previous decades.

Of course these machines and the options they represent are a core component of the ethical conundrums around end of life in America today.

How Corporatization has Impacted Hospitals

The takeover of hospitals by for-profit corporations, now national chains, has had a profound effect on staffing, particularly on nursing. Since nursing is one of hospitals' highest costs, it's not surprising that hospitals would focus cost-cutting efforts on nursing expenditures.

Corporate hospital chains have cast their shadow over all hospitals. In terms of the issues I raise in this book, hospitals are more similar than they are different. All compete for customers from a common pool. If one hospital adds a service or lowers its costs, others are going to follow suit. If one adds family-friendly ethical resources, others will eventually—if not because they want to, then to compete in the marketplace.

The Goal of Hospital Treatment and its Relation to Insurance

In general, the insurance companies pay for treatment. Treatment requires the diagnosis of a treatable condition. The diagnosis is converted to one or more billable treatment codes. If a patient's condition is not or is no longer curable by traditional allopathic medical treatments, the insurance companies won't pay. This means that people don't die of old age in hospitals these days, because old age is not curable and cannot be assigned a diagnostic code, so they are not allowed to stay in the hospital.

Shorter hospitalizations are not necessarily bad. The days of extended hospital stays for other-than-terminal or the most serious conditions are long gone. "Early" discharge from the hospital and going elsewhere (be it rehab or home) can be a good thing. For those with grave conditions requiring extended hospitalization, doctors can usually find an insurance code that will allow them to keep a patient hospitalized for some additional time.

Shorter hospital stays have brought new challenges that didn't exist with longer stays. For example, unless nurses get to know a patient prior to the post-surgical stage, they won't have any frame of reference for how that person responds under normal conditions.

At some point, you must and will be discharged (unless you die). This can become a financial problem when discharge is into long-term rehab, long-term care, or a nursing home. This is because Medicare pays for acute care and for some rehab but not for long-term care. Medicaid, on the other hand, does pay for long-term care, but only for those who qualify because of extreme financial deprivation.

The Effect of Corporate Hospitals on Nursing

If the primary role of hospitalization is to nurse ill patients, what explains the decimation of American nursing? This situation, more than anything, accounts for the enormity of your task as your loved one's personal representative.

Here are some of the ways nursing has changed in response to the corporatization of hospitals:

- Nurse caseloads have steadily increased. Nurses are severely overworked, and new ways are routinely found to try to eke more out of them, all at the expense of patient-family care. For example, after my sister's busy, urban, newborn intensive care unit was downsized by eliminating the secretaries, nurses had to answer the telephone (which rang incessantly) and answer the intercom to buzz parents into the secured unit. They were responsible for premature and critically-ill, full-term newborns on life support in NICU plus a busy well-baby unit, yet had to act as their own receptionists, all while handling growing patient loads, which meant more phone calls and parent visits.
- Individual care has been replaced by a production-line model. Nurse-managers oversee a dwindling number of RNs. Tasks formerly done by nurses are now done by technicians with little

training, a narrow skill set, and less patient contact. Thus, more people spend less time with more patients. This joins the lack of a physician-in-charge in contributing to discontinuity of care.

- Nurses lose seniority if they relocate (either to a different hospital chain within a city or by moving to a new city). They're trapped. Want to move across the country? Even if you're a twenty-year veteran, resign yourself to going back to the night shift and crawling your way out of it again.
- Nurses, no matter their skill, closeness to their patients, or gender, remain subservient to doctors in a class system. The doctors are scientists; nurses want to be healers. Nurses are also the providers who are or have the potential to be closest to their patients. Yet nurses must constantly defer to doctors. All day, every day.

Nurses' Response to Stress and Duress

Some studies have shown that nurses in professionally disenfranchised workplaces engage in serious infighting, to the detriment of patient care (not to mention their own well-being).[44] Their educational curriculum trains them to value and provide care in the way that you and I perceive care, but conditions in their workplace make doing so an ideal that's difficult to meet. This both results from and results in behind-the-scenes friction, a sure way of compromising patient-family treatment.

Nursing Staff Know Less about Their Patients Nowadays

Nurses have less patient contact than in the past. Part of this is because patients spend fewer days hospitalized. If nurses have not experienced your loved one prior to elective surgery or the onset of a medical crisis, they may have no idea of your loved one's healthy state, their level of intellectual competency, or the nature of their responses to stimuli. In other words, they lack a complete view from which to gauge their patient.

Hospital Patients are Sicker than Before

In general, hospital patients are sicker than before. Due to outpatient clinics for a growing number of procedures, plus our ability to manage illness and extend life, we enter hospitals only when something goes seriously wrong. Thus, a higher percentage of nurses' patient load presents as more complex and demanding than in years past.

Several Well-known Hospitalization Risks

POTENTIALLY LIFE-THREATENING ASPECTS of hospitalization are reported ever more frequently. In many reports, they are discussed under the umbrella of "medical mistakes." Primary among them are breaches of hygiene, hospital-borne infection, mislabeled IV fluids, and operating on the wrong part of the body. We experienced the first two.

Breaches of Hygiene and Hospital-borne Infections

Believe it or not, good hygiene is often forgotten, even in the modern-day hospital. During each parent's terminal hospitalization, we observed repeated breaches of hygiene. Utensils and medical equipment like heating pads that had been dropped on the floor were repositioned on the tray or table for future use by our very ill parents. Invariably my sister would catch these breaches, dispose of or dispense with the object in question, and wipe the surface with disinfectant.

Maintaining hygiene is the first line of defense against hospital-borne infection. In recent years The Joint Commission has been trying to rectify this. There should be a wall-mounted container of waterless disinfectant near the room door, and everyone entering the room ought to reflexively dispense and wipe their hands with some of it. Do it yourself, and see to it that everyone else does, too—especially doctors and staff whose day consists of moving from room to room touching patients and the stuff surrounding them. Have the docs wipe off their stethoscopes, too. If there's no dispenser, buy a bottle yourself, place it at the bedside, kindly insist that everybody use it, and set an example by using it yourself.

We have no proof, but Judy and I feel certain that the urinary tract infection my father contracted while hospitalized was hospital-borne; he'd never had a urinary infection during his eighty-four years of life. Infections can and do kill; using the best precautions to prevent them is essential. If, as in Dad's case, the infection is identified as MRSA,[45] extremely strong antibiotics must be administered intravenously.

Mislabeled IV Fluids and Medications

Patients today wear scannable, bar-coded wristbands. All fluids (intravenous drips) and medicines intended for ingestion must be ordered by doctors on the treatment group, assembled and delivered to the room, and administered by nurses. These items will also be bar coded. Read all labels with your own eyes and ensure your loved one's name—correctly spelled—is on them. Refuse to allow any fluid or pill to be administered to your loved one if their labels' name and ID numbers don't match your loved one's exactly, even if a nurse tries to downplay the mismatch.

The Need to Oversee Your Loved One's Treatment

DESPITE DOCTORS' ROLES AS PHYSICIAN-SCIENTISTS, and despite hospital procedures and command/control structure that you'd think would result in careful daily treatment of your loved one, patient-family oversight is required. Many reasons exist for this requirement, including discontinuity of care (described below), bias that sometimes prevents treatment providers from seeing each patient as a unique case whose particulars may differ from other individuals with similar symptoms, occupational arrogance, and systemic incompetence.

No matter the cause, 24/7 oversight is the ideal. Like medical mistakes, the need for family oversight is also well-reported and documented. Such stories typically feature reformed doctors who have finally experienced hospitalization from the vantage point of either being a patient or as personal representative to their hospitalized spouse.

The need for patient advocacy has become unquestioned. Even hospitals suggest having an advocate if you become a patient. It's unfortunate that hospitals are not required to explain *why* patient advocacy is necessary. By answering this question, institutions would be forced to admit how the care they claim to provide has morphed into monitoring that can be inadequate much of the time.

"Family Care" Means Your Family Provides the Care

THE TERM "FAMILY CARE" MAY TAKE ON A NEW MEANING during hospitalization: that your family must care for your loved one beyond the bodily repair services offered by physicians and monitoring provided by nurses.

You're lucky if you have an attentive nurse overseeing your loved one; because, in general, care has been removed from nursing. There's not enough time and not enough nurses to provide it. A skeleton of checkpoints has replaced the body of care we used to expect. There's no more meat on nursing's bones—until you, the previously unsuspecting, now-informed personal representative, appear and assume your role as overseer and impromptu nurse-in-training. The good news is that in some circumstances, if you're good, your loved one's nurses will eventually accept you as part of the treatment group, and you and they will have become partners.

If your loved one cannot feed him- or herself and you are unavailable or uncomfortable doing the feeding yourself, you need to hire outside assistance. The hospital food service personnel merely bring in the food tray at one moment and remove it at another. Your loved one may be sleeping during those times. The nurses might not know if your loved one consumed anything and if not, why not.

This is not the kind of "care" that hospitals admit to providing. Nor is it the type of lapse that makes any nurse proud. Regardless, it occurred over several days' time at an accredited hospital advertising itself as one of the country's "100 Best." Patients going unfed and without water indicates one of two things: that there simply are not enough nurses to provide the quality of oversight that you and I recognize as care, or that hospital protocols were either absent or had been ignored.

The Family-Friendly Hospital Environment

The hospital either makes itself family-friendly or it doesn't. In terms of physical structures, the most likely to be family-friendly are newer facilities and remodeled wings of older facilities. In terms of the necessary institutional support, the most likely to be family-friendly are faith-based institutions which manifest their core charter by including integrative and palliative care options and the more active oversight of critical cases by the ethics group. Community hospitals in comparatively well-off, small cities may offer the same enhancements as faith-based hospitals, but due rather to the social milieu present in the community. Family-friendly hospitals provide:

- Ample and comfortable seating in the patient room
- Overnight sleeping (recliner or pull-out) in the patient room
- Nearby private meeting rooms for treatment conferences
- Nearby private retreat rooms with telephones for families
- A variety of therapies that humanize the environment for patient-families; for example, music, the aroma of unexpected food like popcorn, trained pets on visiting rounds, and short massages.

Neither of the hospital environments my family inhabited during my parents' demise were remotely family-friendly (my mother's intensive care unit was, in practice, anti-family in the extreme, with tightly restricted visitation policies and scornful family treatment). I did learn, much later, that the hospital my father was in had a newly remodeled wing with private meeting rooms for treatment conferences. We were not advised of this and never thought to ask. But you should ask, either for initial placement or a transfer. Your patient-family will feel and perform better in supportive accommodations.

Where Treatment Discussions and Conferences Take Place

Treatment discussions are periodic conversations that occur between one or several doctors and patient-family members. Treatment *conferences* are large team events that will occur behind closed doors, convening the larger treatment group plus some administrative personnel, typically in response to a significant patient-family medical problem or complaint. Both conversations will be intimate.

There's nothing wrong with treatment conferences occurring in the patient's room (assuming that in your culture the patient should be part of the conference). But not all conferences can occur there, and some discussions ought to occur out of earshot of a patient, whether that patient is conscious or not.

In my experience with various physicians on my mother's case, the docs feel in their element any place inside the hospital. Thus, you will end up in deeply personal treatment conference with a doctor wherever the two of you happen to be standing, whether a busy public hallway or a tiny waiting room filled with other families there for the long haul, eating junk food and queued up for the sole telephone,[46] along with the ubiquitous, blasting TV (so much for HIPAA privacy mandates).

I truly would have preferred a supply closet to the halls and waiting rooms for our treatment conferences. Although I conferenced with the docs wherever we happened to be because I needed to talk with them, my internal response to doing so in these environments ranged from unsettling to feeling disrespected to deeply repugnant.

In fairness, doctors are extremely busy people, with responsibility to many, and they may not have the time to trudge to a meeting room at the far corner of a hospital floor. But what if there were meeting rooms centrally located on every wing, a few steps away? Either none existed at the hospitals my parents were in or we weren't told about them.

The fact that doctors feel comfortable conducting intimate conversations in crowded public places does not mean that we are comfortable doing so or that those venues are appropriate or supportive. So before launching into an intricate treatment consultation in public, ask if there's a private conference room available nearby.

Discontinuity of Care and Discontinuity of Communication

CONTINUITY OF CARE HAS TO DO WITH PREVENTING GAPS in the administration and oversight of the treatment a patient receives and the communication of that treatment to the family. In our context, continuity means that a physician with a complete and holistic sense of the case coordinates and makes sense of your loved one's condition as a whole (specialists tend to see and treat the organ of their specialty rather than the person lying in the bed).

Continuity of communication means that medical information is readily available to all treatment group members including you, the personal representative. It further means that every doctor on the case proactively initiates conversations with the patient-family, conveying important medical information and ethical viewpoints.

Attending physicians talk to each other through their own private channels, excluding you. The problem is that no one then communicates with you on a regular, predictable basis.[47] So, unless you're around when the doctors are, your decision-making process slows down, encumbered by the absence of first-hand information. What comes to mind is some bizarre rendition of the old "telephone" game we played as children, where a message goes around a circle of participants and ends up confused and distorted.

Although the game is funny, there's nothing amusing about discontinuity of communication and treatment during a loved one's hospital stay or about playing telephone tag with doctors. Your loved one's condition and treatment are unpredictable enough, due to their own state, the inherent uncertainty of medical outcome, known clinical risks during hospitalization, plus the vagaries of hospital time. It's particularly annoying to never interact with the doctor(s) and, instead, have to seek out nurses to learn what has been written into your loved one's chart by each attending physician.

On the other hand, even nurses contacting your loved one on a monitoring schedule will have more bedside time with them than any single doctor (aside from a lengthy surgery). Nurses remain a steadfast and vital go-to resource to learn about your loved one's condition.

Another contributor to discontinuity of care is the presence of medical specialists who partition treatment, focusing on this or that organ or component system. It is well documented that specialists tend towards tunnel vision, viewing the patient condition primarily (and sometimes solely) through the filter of their own specialty.

Critically ill patients are often in great flux, and a variety of specialists may end up on their case. These docs offer differing prognoses based on the narrow focus of their specialties (this is referred to as "component management"). Knowing how to interpret their assessments and recommendations can be a critical aspect of how you view your loved one's life-and-death choice points. Without continuity of care, no doctor has an overview or can make sense of the whole. Without continuity of communication, neither can you.

Different specialists can order conflicting treatments or stop a treatment another specialist had begun. We may first experience discontinuity of care when we encounter a treatment newly added by one doctor that conflicts with a prior one established by another doctor. Nurses are the people who typically discover these conflicts and engage the doctors about resolving them. Pharmacists also catch these instances where a poor treatment choice is evidenced by prescription orders ranging from questionable to downright dangerous.

Such a system presents nightmares for a personal representative who needs to consult with a single physician in charge to obtain a medically informed overview of this particular patient as a whole human being. Technically, that person is the admitting physician. Without knowing the type and frequency of behind-the-scenes doctor-to-doctor communication, there's no way that personal representatives can assess how actively their loved one's care is being coordinated.

Worse, your overarching patient-family values may be overlooked. If so, you're at the juncture of clinical problems and ethical problems. Medical ethicists with whom I have spoken are in agreement that discontinuity of care is a prevalent problem.

One step some hospitals are taking to try to alleviate discontinuity of care is to hire their own doctors, who round on their own, and in so doing "join" the treatment group. Do not expect the problem to be solved in a hospital that directly employs doctors as *hospitalists*. Hospitalists work on shifts like all other hospital staff, they do not have a formal relationship with your loved one, and each one may need considerable coaching on the intricacies of your case. In some circumstances, adding a hospitalist to the case may be an instance of yet another "cook in the kitchen."

Who Not to Complain To and What to Know if You Do

IF FRUSTRATION WITH HOSPITAL CONDITIONS or your loved one's condition builds, you may decide to engage nursing management at the hospital administrative level. Based on our experiences, I say *don't*—it's useless. They're the wrong people to engage, unless you've gotten to the point of threatening a lawsuit.[48]

> *DURING THE FIRST WEEK OF MOM'S ICU STAY, we became increasingly frustrated with breaches of hygiene, lack of care, overall signs of disinterest, and regulations severely limiting family access to our loved one. Despite our queries and complaints at the nursing station, nothing changed. One morning,*

after some slight, Judy and I had had enough. We marched down to the office of the Director of Nursing. We'd asked for her name at the nursing station, and I was angry about whatever we'd just experienced. The nurses evidently phoned the administration wing that an angry guy was en route; we were intercepted partway by a person who determined I wasn't homicidal and ushered us into administration.

We spent forty-five emotional minutes describing all the problems compromising our mother's care and our experience in the unit. The VP-level nurse clucked over us and exclaimed, "That's not who we are. These are not our values. This does not reflect our mission statement." She promised remedies.

Nothing changed.

Some days later, after a steady dose of the same experiences, Judy and I convened a treatment conference with the full range of nursing staff. We did this without Dad's knowledge, as we didn't want to burden or be overridden by him. In attendance were the nursing director, several ICU nurses including the shift charge nurse, and, to our surprise, a risk manager, who was in this case a hospital lawyer. It was a long meeting. Judy and I were novices at personal representation.

Nothing changed.

During Dad's hospitalization, before I was called on the scene, Judy again attempted to engage nursing management. After discovering that Dad was not being fed, she marched downstairs and attempted to meet with the Director of Nursing. This time she was denied contact and shunted to a staff person.

Engaging management-level people in each of these facilities was a complete waste of time.[49] These conversations produced no remedies, only endurance matches as we described our concerns, protestations that they and their institution wouldn't engage in such substandard activities and procedures, statements of their intention to look into them, promises to correct deficiencies in our loved one's care, and their

unstated ruminations about what sort of legal risk we might
represent.

Nothing changed.

Such is the depth of the disconnect; no straight communication by the institutions and our own stupid, stubborn, wishful inability to see that our understanding of care is not the medical establishment's implementation of care.

I F YOU'RE GOING TO TALK TO THE WRONG PEOPLE on your own, without the benefit of an ethics counselor or patient advocate, here are some things to consider. Note that "outcome" in this discussion has to do with patient-family experience and treatment, not your loved one's health outcome:

- My assessment of the nursing director in charge of Mom's ICU is that she was in deep denial of the reality in her institution. I'll go out on a limb and expand this assessment to any nursing director who asserts that their institution functions from a place of heartfelt caring while allowing patient-family mistreatment to continue (no matter what their mission statement may put forward). Nursing directors' training, like all nurses, emanates from a core goal to provide compassionate care. Corporate hospitals have long since moved away from that service model. The nursing director will not change the institutional culture or the way a unit functions. High-level administrators are keenly aware of their mission statement's contents. Assuming they buy into them, they're between a rock and a hard place when their units do not function accordingly.
- Expect nothing to change, except the possibility of conditions getting worse because you've annoyed one or more of the staff, even if you've been nonabrasive. Note that annoying staff is *not* a valid reason to meekly acquiesce to patient-family mistreatment.
- The first thing to do when opening a gripe meeting or a treatment conference is to state your goals. Have an outcome in mind. State it clearly and up front so that everyone knows the goal of the meeting. Toward the end of the meeting, ask specifically for

the outcome you want. Ask if the outcome is reasonable. Ask what impediments to a remedy exist in the unit. Ask what the hospital will do to ensure the desired outcome. Ask when to expect that outcome and what changes on the floor will indicate that the outcome has occurred. Ask who is responsible for that outcome. Ask who to engage if the outcome fails to materialize. (Ask ask ask; the mantra of an effective personal representative.)

If the above assessment seems harsh, consider the context that would prompt you, as a loved one, to engage nursing management or convene a large-scale treatment conference. We did not take these actions lightly, nor did I reach the above conclusions lightly. We acted only after repeated instances that added up to a pattern that we could no longer tolerate. The questions we had to answer were, "Is our patient-family treatment healing or detrimental?," and, "When is enough enough?"

Who Pays How Much for What?

The discussion of family involvement would be incomplete without at least a token mention of finances. This is yet another huge topic, and I have limited guidance to offer about managing the cost of elder and terminal care, whether end of life or otherwise. However, recognizing its importance for most of us, I can summarize what I've learned during the aftermath of my father's demise.

My parents were fully insured, with Medicare, medical "gap" insurance (in case they became liable for charges beyond what Medicare would cover), and long-term care insurance. Since neither of them exited the hospital, their long-term care insurance went unused. Mom's hospital bill totaled roughly $150,000 gross, and Dad's approximately $85,000 gross. Medicare paid all of the negotiated costs (some net amount, unknown to me, which was less than the bills' face amount) except for about $125 that had squeaked through to the estate. Note that these were hospital costs only; I have never seen and have no idea what all the doctor and specialist costs were (we can speculate they ran to the tens of thousands of dollars).

Had their gap insurance been engaged, my parents would have been responsible for a co-pay. Had a long-term nursing home been required, that would have cost $4,000 to $7,000 per month, with insurance covering roughly half of that ongoing expense.

Key Things about Health Insurance and Hospital Costs

Here are some key things to know regarding health insurance for the aged who are not self-insured:

The federal Medicare program (for seniors and the disabled) pays for acute care and limited rehabilitation. Medicare does not pay for ongoing rehab and does not pay for long-term or nursing home care.

The federal Medicaid program (for the poor) pays for long-term and nursing home care. One must possess virtually no assets in order to qualify. Medicaid is administered on the state and county level.

Disability insurance for those who have not reached Medicare's age of eligibility is delayed for six months from the date one is *approved* by the government (not the date of application). Denied approvals can be contested and usually require a lawyer specializing in doing so, at a cost of about $5,000. Appeals will add three to six months to the application period. Costs during the entire application/approval period are *not* reimbursable.

Private insurance is available, but—as is always the case with insurance—the fewer the pre-existing conditions and the earlier you buy it (before something disqualifies you), the less it will cost and fewer conditions will be excluded from coverage.

If you are insured privately, engage a professional accountant to assist with vetting all the bills. Medical billing is complex and hospital billing is routinely error-prone. If you're self-paying, know that you can negotiate with hospitals for better rates (by default, they bill individual payers a "retail" rate rather than the discounted rate insurers pay).

A legal specialty has evolved around financial issues common to the infirm elderly. Of central concern is how to protect assets without actually utterly depleting them and how to divest oneself of them in order to meet Medicaid's stringent, poverty-inducing eligibility requirement (literally, down to about $3,000 total personal assets). As an example, if you are elderly and have children you can trust with your money and other assets while you're alive, there may be ways to move assets out of your name, still obtain the support and benefits the assets have always provided you, and qualify for Medicaid because technically your assets have been removed from your control.

These are complex legal matters. The expertise required to accomplish them requires a law firm specializing in elder medical-financial affairs. Unless you plan to die at home, and actually do, your wealth can be stripped in short order if you have not undergone comprehensive legal planning for end-of-life healthcare. (And even at-home deaths can be proceeded by years of significant healthcare expenses.)

Family Involvement in Hospital Care Recap: What You Can Do

If your loved one is hospitalized, document everything throughout each day and night. Maintain notes (your personal "chart") or keep a journal.

Be an effective question-asker! *Start now*. Has this chapter answered all your questions about:

- What hospitals have become and why?
- The relationship between treatment options, goals, and insurance?
- The realities, challenges, and limitations of nurses' working environment?
- The importance of good hygiene?
- Various hospitalization risks?
- The role your family must play?
- What constitutes a family-friendly hospital environment and how to try to obtain it?
- Treatment discussions and conferences?
- The relationship between discontinuity of care and discontinuity of communication?
- Who not to complain to?
- The basics of financial responsibility for costs?

If you do not have all the information you need, write your questions down. How will you get them answered? Reread this chapter? Internet research? Library research? Consulting with family and friends? A phone call to a professional or organization? Go online or pick up the phone book, find a likely contact, and send the email or place the call.

5 | Forecasting and Ethical Support: What You Need to Know, When You Need to Know It, and How to Get It

W E WERE AT THE END OF THE LINE—*the intake process for admission to hospice. It was a Friday afternoon. Judy, myself, and a hospice intake nurse were at Dad's bedside. Luckily, the county hospice agency maintained a special wing in the hospital just down the hall from where we'd been, so there was no need for an ambulance trip to some other facility.*

Hospice intake is a careful procedure. A one to two hour-long interview. Multiple forms to complete and re-verify. Questions to answer. The hospice intake nurse ensures the patient-family is lucid and fully understands what they are doing. In our case, the process unfolded over a three-to-four-hour period.

The forms signed, the arrangements made, we kiss and hug Dad and tell him we'll return around dinner time.

Later, with Dad sleeping and settled in for the night, Judy and I leave the unit to consider what's in front of us.

What's in front of us is a grave choice. Our problem: the hospice intake did not address what to do about the various medications Dad was on. Our choice: leave Dad on chemical life support—the daily fistful of heart meds without which his heart would fail—or order them stopped immediately. Keeping him on heart meds would allow for the unlikely miracle of his rebounding from the bladder and wrist infections but otherwise prolong his demise. Stopping his heart meds would preclude any chance of a miracle, since his heart was functioning at only thirty percent of a healthy heart's capacity.

Our conundrum: we imagined Dad awakening, as he did from time to time during his first day in hospice. Only this time he'd have improved—one of the infections would miraculously be in remission. He'd be better, brighter. No longer out of it. And I would have to look at my father and say, "Dad, I decided to stop your heart meds two days ago."

Over the weekend, Judy and I anguished over a decision we never expected to have to make…after all, our parents had engaged in advance planning. They had executed a full suite of Power Documents, and we had had family conversations around the dining room table, reviewing their wishes.

This was needless duress; with adequate forecasting, it would not have been necessary.

FOR THOSE IN ACUTE NEED OR CRISIS

YOUR PATIENT-FAMILY NEEDS TIMELY COMMUNICATION about how the institution functions, your loved one's condition, possible changes in it, and what you might need to contemplate before the next foreseen choice point arrives with a requirement that you make a decision. Ethicists call this FORECASTING.

Forecasting is the communication of things most vital for a patient-family to know. What we're told and when we're told it are equally vital.

With forecasting, our emotional upheaval, although potentially great, is kept to a minimum. WITHOUT FORE-CASTING, UNNECESSARY AND DISRUPTIVE SHOCK WILL BE ADDED TO OUR BURDEN. This shock is intellectual, emo-tional, physical, and spiritual. It will interfere with your ability to make decisions and your loved one will languish until you recover from the shock.

For help obtaining forecasting and with making these most difficult decisions, look for two resources: the right patient liaison (if you have a choice, the best is an RN -- a registered nurse -- due to his or her clinical knowledge) and a full-time hospital chaplain. FIND THESE PEOPLE BEFORE YOU NEED THEM. Ask them to check in on you daily. Their presence in an institution is a sign of at least some orientation toward patient-family support. Their absence is cause for concern.

Modern chaplains ought to be open-minded, multifaceted, non-medical employees who, by virtue of their presence in a hospital, mix easily with doctors and are skilled at negotiating medical treatment problems. If need be, a chaplain (or you) can ask for a consult with the ethics committee -- a request typically reserved for life-and-death circumstances in which you and the treatment group are in deep disagreement.

The Significance of Forecasting and the Shock of its Absence

DURING EACH OF MY PARENTS' DEMISE, the communication most vital to my family was inadequate to make decisions without unnecessary additional shock. The vital communication was, by turns, withheld, incomplete, or delayed by days—days during which the family could have come to grips with looming choices that would have accompanied the communication, had it occurred.

The communication we lacked is known in healthcare ethics as *forecasting*. Do not expect doctors and nurses to know or use this term, although once exposed to it they'll readily understand its meaning.

To forecast means to advise of and estimate future events. Prognosis, while technically a synonym for forecasting, is understood to refer to a rather specific health outcome (e.g., Will she recover or remain afflicted? Will he live or die?). In the hospital, future events include not only your loved one's ultimate outcome, but how things proceed during hospitalization, possible choice points along the way, and when various events will, or are likely to, occur. In the hospital environment, prognosis is a subset of forecasting.

The term is attributable to the medical ethicist Diann B. Uustal, RN, MS, EdD, from whom I first heard it.[50] In the medical ethics community, forecasting occurs during treatment discussions and treatment conferences ranging from informal, on-the-spot talks between the patient and a doctor to sit-down events, with a large number of treatment group and family members.

In my experience, forecasting is among the most critical type of communications. It contains the most vital content and, aside from treatment details, is the only communication you're really interested in when your loved one's remaining days may be counted on your fingers.

I've extended Uustal's definition of forecasting, broadening the universe of future events to include disclosure about how the institution functions and how you, as the personal representative, can function most effectively within it, e.g., about situations which you are likely to encounter. Forecasting considers both what is likely to happen and what could possibly happen if the patient takes a turn for the worse. To avoid extrinsic shock, we must know what to be ready for if the treatment plan fails; what decisions might conceivably be required several days from this moment.

How might this look in terms of communication with family members? An attending physician might say something like this: "The treatment path we're on aims to restore your loved one to ABC level of biomechanical functioning. It will take four to five days to ascertain this. At that point, two outcomes are possible. Outcome 1 would require us all to consider UVW; outcome 2 would require that we all consider XYZ. Since XYZ is dire, you may want to give outcome 2 some thought during the next few days. Please consider the issues, so if outcome 2 arises, you will all be ready, at that time, to choose what to do about it."

Is committing time and energy to mulling over a possible outcome several days from now a waste of time? Yes and no. In the workaday world, perhaps conjecture is a time-waster. During a terminal hospitalization, conjecture equates to advance planning. If you don't conjecture and your loved one's condition worsens, s/he may languish while you and your family take in new, shocking information and then parse decisions. Having spent agonizing days parsing life-and-death decisions, I can tell you that I'd rather conjecture and be ready to move as soon as a choice point is reached, rather than subject my loved one to several more days of languishing, most likely in discomfort if not in outright pain.

Forecasting is critical. I've experienced the repeated lack of it, and on that basis I say it forms a baseline of care for the patient-family; that without forecasting, care is compromised and incomplete. Forecasting should provide help in making weighty healthcare decisions. With forecasting, you will know, generally, what to expect. Without forecasting, you are subject to surprise. Shock, actually, is the experience.

Of course, it is the family who will be shocked. Unless the patient's condition nosedives, medical practitioners will not be shocked at all; they've trod these paths time and again.

Intrinsic and Extrinsic Shock

I introduced intrinsic and extrinsic shock earlier under "New Terms for a Clear Conversation." Intrinsic shocks originate from your loved one's condition—the plain fact that your loved one is hospitalized, takes a turn for the worse, or the specter of their dying. Extrinsic shocks originate from sources outside the family, typically due to inadequacies in how treatment proceeds during hospitalization.

The specter of a loved one in serious or life-threatening medical condition is shocking. If it's occurring without notice, that's another layer of shock. If you've hastily flown cross-country and are a personal representative with life-and-death decision-making responsibility, if you've got dysfunctional family dynamics, if you're AWOL from work or in financial need, these circumstances equate to additional layers of intrinsic shock.

Intrinsic shock goes with this territory. Ideally, the system's treatment of its patient-family customers would exhibit care, to help buffer and support the patient-family. While care may occur occasionally, our experiences were of cold systems that provided patient treatment and periodic oversight, but essentially abandoned the family (and to an extent, the patient) for various periods of time, leaving them in their own uninformed bubble of existence.

That bubble is a breeding ground for extrinsic shock. Because, eventually, the bubble bursts. Perhaps a doctor makes an unexpected announcement, and what the family hoped was curable is pronounced incurable. Perhaps the family believes that the treatment group is aware of the family's advance planning documents and that the boundaries they discuss are in effect, only to learn that neither is the case. Perhaps what the family has considered to be a simple black-and-white directive suddenly becomes gray, murky, mired in ethical considerations that have never been introduced to them.

These conditions, in and of themselves, are not the cause of extrinsic shock. Rather, it's their abrupt communication that causes unnecessary shock for the family. Unnecessary because, in the hospital, possibilities are well known and can be shared, sometimes days in advance. As one example of forecasting's role, when possibilities are forecast, people have the forewarning required to examine, discuss, and come to grips with them.

You will experience extrinsic shocks as particularly acute. To some degree, you will have already begun accepting your loved one's condition, and several days into a hospitalization you will have settled into some sort of routine (probably not comfortable, but predictable, within certain parameters).

"Acute," as a medical term, means "having a sudden onset, sharp rise, and short course." According to the online dictionary MedicineNet.com, acute "also connotes an illness that is rapidly progressive and in need of urgent care."

We who suffer the acute effects of extrinsic shock require some urgent care. At the least, these shocks interfere with our equilibrium. At the worst they cause angst, cost time and effort, and diminish our effectiveness as personal representatives.

Shock due to a lack of forecasting is not merely injurious in the abstract; it's injurious in fact. It's experienced as an emotional thunderclap. Extrinsic shock stuns. It impairs and delays our ability to assess clearly and make decisions. But unlike intrinsic shock, extrinsic shock emanates from the system and is, in most cases, completely avoidable.

I'll provide case examples of extrinsic shock from my family experiences in "The Complete Do-Not-Resuscitate Conversation." At this point, suffice it to say that shock suffered by patients or families due to lack of forecasting is, in my experience, malpractice. This means "bad practice," defined by Webster as "injurious." It's not malpractice in the sense that you'd sue over it, but I use this highly charged word to make the point that extrinsic, avoidable shock administered in the healthcare sector is harmful and violates the fundamental medical ethic to first do no harm.[51] *Extrinsic shock is harmful.*

If providers viewed their customer as the patient-family, the do-no-harm ethic would extend to the treatment of family members actively involved in providing care in the hospital, or at the *very* least the patient and designated POA. Hospitalization now requires oversight by and involvement of family members who advocate for their loved one (which actually means to protect a loved one from clerical, nursing, and medical mistakes). The very notion of patient advocacy equates to an admission that patients are at systemic risk when hospitalized. The family is thus required to fill a void resulting from systemic failures, including too few nurses to actually "nurse" (distinct from monitor) their patients. But the system, in general, habitually treats families as outsiders by not treating them at all (at best) and mistreating them (at worst).

My use of the term *administered* makes it seem like the shock is the result of something purposefully provided (or at least not purposefully *avoided*), rather than as the result of things forgotten or overlooked. I use it intentionally. I cannot believe that this country's physicians, highly intelligent scientists who have put themselves through ten to fifteen years of arduous training, whose *chosen* field revolves around daily intimate human contact, cannot evaluate their own behavior and implement humane protocols. I conclude, therefore, that they have chosen to ignore doing so.

Using the Term *Forecasting*

At this writing, it seems that only ethicists use "forecasting." I've expanded Uustal's definition of forecasting because it seems apt to do so. Members of pastoral care departments seem comfortable with the term without explanation. However, several nurses and an ED physician I questioned report that neither they nor their peers use the term, nor do other hospital personnel recognize it. However, they did immediately understand and seem comfortable with my meaning, once I described it.

If you use "forecasting" in conversation and a treatment provider says, "Huh?", try expanding it into a phrase such as "provide explanations about how things work and when we next need to make a choice, so we can use the intervening time to deliberate and plan in advance."

Forecasting Versus Prognosis

Making prognoses can be tricky business. No doctor (or patient-family) has a crystal ball. It's unreasonable to expect exact predictions from the treatment group regarding the timing of natural processes and their outcomes. Patients can turn on a dime for better or worse. Their progress or demise is almost always stated in terms of probabilities and unknowns.

However, because the treatment plan is less "care" and more "bodily repair under the direction of independent physician-scientists," much is known by the treatment group about the patient's condition—it's likely that the treatment group has already dealt many times before with whatever ails your loved one. Thus, it's reasonable to expect forecasting regarding upcoming choice points and their possible timetable (the latter especially if everyone is waiting for the patient's physiology to respond one way or another to some intervention).

On one hand, prognoses are often inaccurate as evidenced by the fact that people with a poor medical prognosis can recover completely, and people with a favorable prognosis can suddenly worsen and die. On the other hand, in many cases patients follow known trajectories, and when enough aspects of their condition conform to these trajectories, the treatment group's prognosis may be less prescient and simply the product of prior experience.

In any case, do not expect absolute pronouncements from the treatment group. Do expect to have to thoroughly examine all of the philosophical and ethical aspects on your own. In order to do so without extrinsic shock, you merely need some advance notice that it might be prudent to do so.

List of Questions to Have Answered on the Front End

To effectively represent your loved one, you need to know how things work in a hospital. Unless you want to learn the hard way, with no time to think, it's important to have as much information up front as possible.

Here's a list of things that you will want to know at the outset. Having acquired answers to these issues through countless surprises, I can say that knowing the following—up front—results in an easier hospitalization and more effective patient representation:

- Does any part of the hospital provide a family-friendly environment (examples include sleeping quarters for family in the patient room; meeting rooms for treatment conferences; access to communication resources such as a library, telephone, and the internet)? If some part of the building has been remodeled and includes family-friendly resources, ask that your loved one be admitted to or transferred to that wing.
- Are there "concierge" types of services that support family comfort, such as meals or a stash of soft drinks and snack foods, or massages?

- Are there gaps in nursing service that you may want to fill (personally or with personally hired, outside helpers who come to the hospital)?
- Which of your loved one's advance planning documents have been submitted and enacted? (Remember that these steps are distinctly different.)
- What are the relevant policies and routines, including times and reasons for family exclusions from patient contact and from the premises?
- What time do the doctors visit patients (called "rounding" or "making their rounds")?
- What are the doctors' relationships with the hospital and with one another? Which doctors are independent with privileges to practice within the hospital, which doctors are "hospitalists" employed by the hospital, and which doctor is in fact in charge of your loved one's overall case?
- What is the range of providers who will attend to your loved one and how do you identify them—for example, how do you differentiate registered nurses (licensed in comprehensive assessment, intervention, and care) from lower-level nurses and from technicians (the latter being quickly and narrowly trained to perform a distinct task)?
- What is the range of providers who may operate on your loved one and what are each of their roles in the operating room?
- Who else may be present in the operating room and why?
- Who is responsible for determining whether your loved one's insurance coverage(s) apply to each individual providing services?
- What are the intervals between treatment events and choice points that require decisions?
- How are weekends and holidays staffed and how does this affect treatment delivery and options? (Note: *it shouldn't.*)
- What is the range of general patient conditions that might reasonably develop during hospitalization, based on the patient particulars (age, condition, reason for arrival)?

- What potential ethical conundrums might arise and what procedures are available to families to contest decisions they disagree
  with, especially when critical life-and-death outcomes are at
  stake and quick or immediate response is required?
- What institutional measures are in place to combat hospital-
  borne infections? What are the hygiene practices that all staff
  must adhere to?

A daunting list? Absolutely. Welcome to hospitalization, where many
important issues require your oversight.

If you're wondering when and how you can get these questions
answered, let me suggest that you don't try before you have first taken
time to commune with your loved one, settle in, and get over the shock
(at least slightly) of being in the hospital. Then, realize that you've entered
a unique time zone, *hospital time* (which we'll examine in the next chapter). There will be many periods of waiting. Use those periods to obtain
answers to these questions. Bit by bit, the pieces will fall into place.

The Need for Forecasting on the Back End, Too

My sister and I, co-medical powers of attorney during our father's
demise, agonized for that weekend over an end-of-life directive. It turned
out our agony was completely unnecessary. It could have been rendered
moot with a little inquiry and forecasting during Dad's intake procedure.

*JUDY AND I FELT LIKE WE HELD THE LAST HOPE for our father's
life in our hands.[52] It was heartbreaking. We agonized and
finally decided that the miracle was unlikely. We girded ourselves to march into hospice early Monday morning to meet
the hospice doc as he rounded and fight for stopping all of
Dad's meds. We remained burdened and tense throughout
the weekend.*

*Monday morning came. It turned out that the hospice doc
agreed with us. He did us one better, saying, "Some of these
meds are actually palliative; they'll provide comfort for him.
Let's leave Mort on these and stop the rest." It was ordered,
charted, and done. Given that his heart could not function at*

thirty percent capacity without chemical intervention, we knew
that Dad would die a peaceful death within several days' time.

But why were Judy and I, the authorized personal representatives, left to languish and anguish over a life-and-death issue for a night, let alone a weekend? Why did we suffer a complete lack of forecasting even into this very last stage? Why wasn't the patient's medication history evaluated during hospice intake, especially since the patient was alert and available during the several hours that intake required? Why didn't Judy or I think to pursue this ourselves during the hospice intake?

The only answer I have to these questions is that the system failed. The institutions comprising the system failed. This includes the hospital, the hospice, the treatment group members, and we adult children/caretakers.

Note that none of these last-phase failures impacted our father; he was quietly dying, in whatever state of being the dying inhabit. The failures, however, had a massively negative impact on the family.

Final Forecasting Comments

The hospital that hangs a street-side banner reading, "We Forecast Early and Often" would be a strong candidate for my business, other criteria being equal.[53] This would be nicely augmented by posting a sign in every patient room and common area saying, "If you find yourself in decision paralysis, dial H-E-L-P for compassionate help." Doing so would trigger the active involvement of the hospital's family support services—hospital employees who specialize in providing practical and ethical assistance to patients and their families.

Ethical Support Services to Assist with Forecasting

A FAMILY-FOCUSED MEDICAL ENVIRONMENT is, first and foremost, an orientation to and commitment by hospital administrations to value the family half of its patient-family customer base. Acknowledging the role families play would be a good starting point. The next step would be to require that each admitted patient be assigned a lead doctor and that all members of the treatment group have an efficient communication infrastructure facilitating good communication with the lead doctor. Hospitals would inform patients about how they function, why certain treatment steps take a long time to play out, and the sort of ethical dilemmas that arise around certain types of family directives, as well as issues related to resuscitation. They would tell us, up front, about the range of patient-family support services available, how to access them, and what each could do for us. They would also disclose what sort of presence and effort was required of the family to fill the gaps inherent in hospitalized treatment in order to provide the care that the system in its current state is unlikely to provide its patients.

The ideal institution for your loved one would provide a family-friendly environment, a patient liaison, one or more full-time hospital chaplains with staff, and an available, empowered ethics committee—all resources we will learn about next.

Unless and until this ideal is met, we will have to develop a sensitivity to and express our own need of forecasting and ethical support. The balance of this chapter discusses finding ethical support in the hospital: how to determine if it exists, its extent, and the key people who may be employed behind the scenes, ready to help if you should call.

With or without forecasting, a time may come when the treatment group and you—your loved one's personal representative—have different ideas about the proper course of treatment. You may have a conflict to resolve.

Medical providers are highly aware of modern ethical conundrums. Now, in the twenty-first century, the end of life is filled with ethical decisions. The Terri Schiavo case was a highly publicized example. Whatever the details may be in your family's case, I can almost guarantee that your experience will feel as extraordinary and painful, with the full gamut of emotion and ethical soul-searching, as the Schiavo case seemed from the outside—unless you and your loved one have come to terms with dying and death.

Should an impasse develop regarding your loved one's treatment, it's time to enlist the help of trained ethical specialists. An impasse could arise due to insufficient information from the treatment group to support decision-making, a quandary you find yourself in despite having information, or differences of opinion regarding treatment.

Actually, if forecasting is provided to the patient-family, it's likely that no impasse will develop, or that everyone will be alert to a looming impasse and take proactive steps to deal with it, potentially sparing the patient-family days of turmoil (and easing the treatment group's experience as well).

Ethical assistance is invaluable even if—especially if—an impasse is contained within your own heart, mind, and soul.

Because forecasting is an intrinsic part of ethical care, the two are bound together. Thus, as we proceed to explore ethical resources, I will continue to frame them within the context of forecasting.

What Constitutes an Ethical Environment

Before examining specific resources that ought to be available for all hospitalized patient-families, I need to explain what the phrase "ethical environment" means.

Ethics has to do with a code of moral principles. Acting ethically refers essentially to doing what is right. My use of the phrase "ethical environment" regarding hospitals refers to a workplace in which management and practitioners include ethicists as resources to help everybody involved determine what the right thing is in each instance.

The absence of an ethical environment does not mean or imply that hospital management and practitioners do wrong or unethical things. It means only that the institution has not engaged ethicists or made them available to the patient-family. While doctors and family members may have differences of opinion regarding treatment plans and goals, it's clear that doctors provide treatment according to an honest interpretation of their medical oath in a context that is the logical outgrowth of their years of medical training.

An ethical conundrum arises when the patient-family's definition of what constitutes "harm" differs from the practitioners' definition, or when a different set of values is used to make decisions about prolonging life. The most classic examples are those in which a family's values include the full picture, accounting for personhood and quality-of-life issues, while the treatment group's criteria are comparatively narrow, focusing on whether or not the patient's particular organ can survive a particular disease phase during a particular hospitalization and extend the patient's quantity of life regardless of quality.

Forecasting and Ethical Support: Printed Materials

While printed materials themselves do not provide ethical support, they are often a hospital's first attempt to provide notice that ethical support exists at the institution. Printed materials may be provided at admission. While written notice of these services is probably required, pages in a patient handbook or even a separate brochure are not an ideal way to communicate. The patient's agent (the person named in their Medical Power of Attorney) may not arrive on the scene until days after admission and may not encounter or even be aware of the materials. Even if made aware of brochures, the last thing you're likely to do upon arrival is to sit around reading hospital literature.

In any case, be on the lookout for printed materials describing ethical resources. If you don't see them, ask for them.

Forecasting and Ethical Support: The Need to Ask

You are unlikely to find notice of any forecasting services. I suspect that this is because the system assumes adequate communication by providers as part of treatment management. The adequacy of information provided may vary. Some nurses are particularly attentive, and some are rushed and harried. Remember that most doctors are independent of the hospitals in which they round. Some doctors will give you advance notice of possible outcomes, and some won't. All are averse to dashing your hope; if you want to know a reasonable range of outcomes as soon as providers know or suspect them, you'll have to explicitly ask each treatment group member to provide it for you.

Forecasting and Ethical Support: The Patient Liaison or Patient Advocate

A patient liaison acts as a communication bridge between the patient-family and medical personnel. In my experience, the patient liaison may simply appear sometime and introduce him- or herself.

What a patient liaison doesn't tell you may be highly important, so you'll have to ask, "What is your professional background?" I've discovered four backgrounds and types of advocates thus far: the specialist liaison, social worker, registered nurse, and case manager.

These professionals have different kinds of training and, therefore, different levels of implicit authority. Authority is important should an ethical conundrum arise, because people tend to dismiss those whose authority is less than their own. In the hierarchical, command/control hospital environment, registered nurses, MDs, and administrators rank higher than a specialist liaison or a social worker.

Specialist Liaison

A specialist liaison may be employed by practices such as orthopedics, where post-operative care is more straightforward than that required during hospitalizations that are (or turn) terminal. A specialist liaison's training will be narrow in comparison to other patient liaisons' training. This person's chief role may be simply to facilitate communication and look in on a patient during post-op rehab.

Social Worker

A social worker, despite what knowledge s/he acquires as a result of working in the hospital, is not medically trained. A social worker may be skilled in understanding the system and in relating to people and advocating for their needs; however, since social workers don't have medical training, doctors, nurses, and hospital administrators may not view a person with this background as an equal. According to a hospital mission director I interviewed, social workers tend to side with families (or are viewed that way by most providers). If medical personnel pigeonhole a liaison as biased, the ability of the liaison to advocate on behalf of a patient-family may be compromised.

Registered Nurse

A registered nurse (RN) who's moved into the role of patient liaison has the benefit of extensive medical training and experience. S/he talks the talk and may be accepted as a colleague by treatment group members. A nurse will be familiar with many aspects of hospitalization and disease trajectory that can result in ethical conundrums, including those initially hidden to families. A registered nurse has the potential to be a strong and sensible advocate.

Case Manager

A case manager is likely to be a management-level hospital employee. This could be good or bad. If you consider hospital management as an adversary, you might prefer an RN as your patient liaison. A management-level patient liaison can be helpful in cases where problems need management attention and buy-in for resolution. The case manager can, for example, deal with a unit manager as an administrative equal. If the case manager is mission-empowered by the hospital administration and if s/he says "we've got a problem to solve," then it's possible that their management-level position will capture the attention of those who must implement the solution. For this reason, one mission director I interviewed feels that case manager patient advocates are an improvement over the others.

This scenario requires that providers and hospital management be alerted to your case and problem. How will this happen? One answer lies in the hospital's pastoral care department and the people who inhabit it.

Forecasting and Ethical Support: The Hospital Chaplain

The pastoral care department is the domain of hospital chaplains. The single most surprising thing my research uncovered is that a full-time hospital chaplain has the keys to the information kingdom in regards to an institution's ethical orientation and resources. This is *the* person you want to find and query.

The dictionary defines *chaplain* as a clergyman officially attached to an institution. As in the military, the hospital chaplain's role is broader than representing a religion or even several religions. Today's best hospital chaplains will be highly trained, skilled resources to help patient-families, doctors, and staff resolve ethical conundrums. My research indicates that you can expect chaplains in medium-to-large metropolitan hospitals to be broad in outlook. None I interviewed acted dogmatically, and all exhibited palpable humanity.

This bears repeating for those for whom the name "chaplain"

connotes a priest who espouses religious dogma. To be sure, chaplains are religious leaders whose role includes ministering to those who so desire. And doubtless some chaplains may espouse strict religious doctrines. The chaplains we're interested in finding view their role as ethical consultants. In a hospital that has formalized its ethical outreach, you will find the chaplain to be a warm and knowledgeable ally. It's imperative to find out, because, when necessary, this person can unlock what one ethicist calls the hospital's "embedded subculture"[54]: ethical experts who understand the issues we face, including the gaps left by doctors and the hospital in patient-families' day-to-day experience.

Hospital chaplains are expert communicators, knowledgeable about medical and ethical matters and skilled in helping people resolve difficult issues. Chaplains ply the institutional back roads that are unmapped for patient-families. They already have the trust, and can gain the attention, of the full cast of characters populating those byways. As per Mark Meaney in *3 Secrets Hospitals Don't Want You to Know: How to Empower Patients*, people accessible to chaplains who are not typically available to patient-families range upward to the hospital risk manager, a high-level administrator consulting directly with the hospital's executive officers.

The first question to ask a hospital chaplain is, "Are you a full-time hospital employee?" If not, that means that chaplains come in, from outside the hospital on some sort of rotating basis.[55] The mission of these outside chaplains will be to minister to patients and families. They may not have the training, expertise, or authority to navigate clinical ethical conundrums or to know their way around the institutional hierarchy.

Religiously based hospitals may have a formal mission department. The director of mission at a metropolitan Catholic hospital advised me that it takes a full year to bring a priest or rabbi off the street and train that individual to function competently in the hospital/medical environment, where many disciplines intersect.

The absence of a full-time hospital chaplain from an institution may indicate something very important: the absence of a management-sanctioned, family-focused, ethical environment.

When a hospital decides to invest resources in developing a family-focused environment to supplement its bodily repair services,

I suspect that its executives will look for people with big hearts who know how to communicate and help: their social workers, nurses, and chaplains (these are the people representing ethics committees that I interacted with). The full-time chaplain will likely know everything about the ethical environment at the institution, because s/he will have been a key participant, perhaps the leader, in its development. Ask, ask, ask questions of the chaplain. Make an hour appointment or take him (or her) to lunch. Chances are you will have a very illuminating and perhaps pointed conversation. The conversation may even prove to be delightful because of the relief it provides, even in the face of a loved one's dire prospects—actually, especially in light of a loved one's dire prospects.

Forecasting and Ethical Support: The Ethics Committee

The ethics committee is a cross-disciplinary group who typically volunteer to serve. They are available to hospital staff and patient-families to examine ethical disputes and suggest resolutions. An ethics committee cannot direct doctors to do or not do one thing or another. The committee can help people try to resolve differences and come to consensus regarding the continuance, cessation, or details of treatment.

Typical ethics committee membership will include one or more of the following people: a patient representative, chaplain, social worker, nurse, doctor, clergy, layperson, and hospital risk manager.

A fledgling ethics committee my be understaffed and little respected by treatment group members. As it develops and matures, interesting things begin to happen. The committee becomes populated with a number of individuals who have studied and earned degrees in clinical bioethics—people who are familiar with the intersection of social, medical, legal, spiritual, and religious issues in a hospital environment. A mature ethical committee will have one or several members available by telephone on a 24/7 basis.

A mature ethical environment is one in which the ethics committee is chartered and championed by hospital administration. Its presence as a resource to both clinicians and families will be well advertised, and clinicians will value the committee as a professional peer group.

Forecasting and Ethical Support Summary

TAKE HEED OF MY EXPERIENCE and do better than we did. Midway through my father's hospitalization, I was approached by a patient liaison who introduced herself and gave me her card. Ironically, I was more jaded toward hospitals then than I am now, so even as I thanked her, I dismissed her as a hospital employee incapable, by the fact of her hospital employment, to offer any useful assistance to us.

What lay behind my dismissal of this person? Here were the questions that went rapid-fire through my mind, which I ought to have asked her outright:

- Why is the hospital paying for a patient advocate?
- If problems occur here that require a patient advocate, what kind of place is this?
- How have you successfully advocated for patients in the past? What were the situational problems, and how were they resolved?[56]

I was wrong in dismissing her. Late in my research, more than a year after Dad died, I called her and we spoke for over an hour. During that conversation, I discovered that she was an RN and could potentially have helped the family navigate some of the problems we experienced during Dad's hospitalization and demise, including the one that resulted in our ceasing curative treatment and moving Dad to hospice, where he died four days later.

During our conversation, she discovered that she hadn't made a strong impression on me and, at her request, I suggested specific things she might say to people when she introduced herself—statements that might have captured my attention had she said them to me.

As a result of my research, I can answer the first two questions I posed above. Patient advocacy has been instituted by hospitals to help bridge the gap between emerging medical ethics and existing institutional inclinations and habits—the gap brought on by technology that lets us push death further and further back in our lives. A gap so significant that bridging it involves the overlapping attention of numerous interests and disciplines including medicine, healthcare, ethics, anthropology, religion, and spirituality. Patient advocates work in places (hospitals) where a variety of interests compete.

ULTIMATELY, IT MATTERS LITTLE WHO YOU FIND TO help you through these ethical problems, whether life and death or not. Although I would gravitate toward those with higher levels of training, I can't say that a person with less training could not help resolve problems. Each hospital is different, and your patient-family circumstances will be unique. In any case, learning about the ethical environment is among the very first things I recommend you do upon your arrival at the hospital. Start with printed materials and, before too much time elapses, get on the telephone. Locating the best people to add to the treatment group, before you even need them, could make a profound difference in how your patient-family experiences the hospitalization. Their presence has the potential to effect your loved one's outcome as well as your overall family experience of their hospitalization. The difference could be huge, in real-time and in your memories.

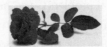

Forecasting and Ethical Support Recap: What You Can Do

If your loved one is hospitalized, document everything throughout each day and night. Maintain notes (your personal "chart") or keep a journal.

Be an effective question-asker! *Start now.* Has this chapter answered all your questions about:

- What comprises forecasting and what may happen without it?
- What you need to know and when you need to know it?
- How shock is inherent in these emergency medical situations and how it can be avoided?
- How to locate family support services in the hospital?
- The various professionals who may appear in ethical support roles and the differences among them?
- The role of the pastoral care department in a modern hospital?

If you do not have all the information you need, write your questions down. How will you get them answered? Reread this chapter? Internet research? Library research? Consulting with family and friends? A phone call to a professional or organization? Go online or pick up the phone book, find a likely contact, and send the email or place the call.

6 | Who's Where, When, Why, for How Long, and Other Turns through the Hospital Maze

D
AD, JUDY, AND I HAD MADE THE DECISION *on a Friday morning to abandon curative treatment—which would have taken the form of an operation on Dad's wrist to drain an infection which had apparently lodged there— and for Dad to enter hospice. His death within some days was a foregone conclusion. Moving him would be easy: the county hospice had located a branch inside the hospital. The intake procedure took three to four hours (interspersed with waiting) and was accomplished by mid-afternoon. We bid Dad goodbye, expecting that his move from the unit room to the hospice wing would take some additional hours. Judy went to collapse and nap in her hotel room, and I returned to Dad's assisted living apartment an hour away to continue doing all the things associated with a terminal hospitalization and its aftermath. We planned on returning to hospice at dinner time to check in on him.*

Shortly after I arrived at the apartment, the phone rang, and the floor nurse advised me that Dad had declared he was not going to hospice without a consult with his admitting physician. Apparently he'd decided to seek her opinion. This made sense to me, even though the anesthesiologists' refusal to oper-

ate according to Dad's no-intubation stipulation left us with no other choices.

I called Judy, waking her up, and made the hour-long drive back to the hospital. She and I met on the unit hallway and, after some animated grousing about Dad's vacillation, we entered his room.

He was absolutely within his rights to request a consult; no argument there. His life was on the line. But the doc had not called back. It was almost five p.m. on a Friday. We had cancelled his hired assistance. Neither Judy nor I could be there all weekend, 24/7.

Judy called Dad's doctor's office. She had to verbally browbeat the doctor's staff to get to the doctor, who gruffly took the call. Only when Judy explained that Dad, facing a life-and-death decision, wanted a final consult with his primary and admitting physician did she take his call.

"But you're my doctor..." he lamented once he got her on the phone.

I will never forget this episode. Had we not broken through the quagmire of indifference shown by Dad's doctor and the hostility of her staff, either Dad might have languished needlessly and painfully over the weekend while awaiting that final consult, or he would have proceeded to hospice without the closure of a final conversation with his primary doctor. Not that the call seemed particularly satisfying; from overhearing Dad's side, we had no indication that this doctor engaged him in an examination of any alternatives to abandoning treatment, much less commiserated with him as a human being.

This situation, along with a vaguely similar one I encountered with Dad's lawyer, impelled me, after Dad's passing, to write both of them a letter scolding them for their absences during critical moments.

I pondered whether or not to send those letters, aware of the irony that my father had forged cordial relationships with *these professionals, with whose services he was happy (he would not have retained them had he been dissatisfied), yet I wound up exhorting them to show up for their patient-family. Why? Discontinuity of care in each case, with the addition of the lawyer failing to recognize that client service to someone who is terminal includes the client's surviving representative, especially when the survivor lives across the country and is trying to accomplish legal business in a limited time frame before returning home.*

FOR THOSE IN ACUTE NEED OR CRISIS

HOSPITALS SEEM to run within a unique time zone I call HOSPITAL TIME. Hospital time determines why there is so much waiting, why some days seem to be devoid of services, when the doctors appear, and other mystifying events explained in this chapter.

BE AT THE BEDSIDE WHEN DOCTORS ROUND -- it's your only chance to talk with them face to face. Typically, rounds occur between 6:30-9 a.m., before office hours. Check with each attending physician to be sure. Know when the docs go off rotation, staying in their office and sending their partners on rounds.

Part of the waiting involves the time it takes for a body's metabolism to respond to medical interventions. Be prepared to cool your jets for 2-4 days, and understand that your loved one's condition may rise and fall during that time. ASK the doctors how long the expected interval will be and WHAT YOU WILL NEED TO DECIDE AT THE NEXT CHOICE POINT.

Try your best to make sure that events scheduled for Thursday or Friday actually occur. Otherwise, chances increase that nothing will occur for another 2-4 days

except your patient-family languishing until the start
of the next workweek.

A range of nurses, technicians, and staff attend
patients. Learn their positions and the range of procedures they are licensed to perform.

You have the right to "fire" providers for unpleas-
antries ranging from bad practice, misrepresentation
(intentional or not), abuse, or irreconcilable differences.
This includes the hospital itself. Know your rights; read
the hospital patient's rights publications (brochure and
lobby placard).

Hospital Time

THE PASSAGE OF TIME AND YOUR EXPERIENCE OF IT take on a new dimension during hospitalizations. I call this phenomenon *hospital time*. Hospital time is characterized by:

- Intervals spent waiting for your loved one's body to respond to medical intervention
- Inexplicable delays in the implementation of doctors' orders
- Delays in the initiation and administration of tests and surgeries
- Doctors making their rounds ("rounding") very early in the morning
- Staffing changes due to recurring calendar dates, including a general slowdown due to weekends and holidays, and potentially riskier periods when new interns flood an institution.

The Time it Takes for a Body to Respond

The body requires time to assimilate treatment and respond to it.

The reasons for problems, or a general decline in your loved one's condition, may not be evident to you and may not even be known by the doctors. In order for doctors to reach a diagnosis, they must consider various likelihoods and test for them. Tests must be scheduled, performed, and analyzed. Then the doctor(s) must order treatment. Due to the body's requirements, in many instances some days must pass before anyone can assess whether or not the treatment has been effective.

Delays Implementing Doctors' Orders

I am not certain why the delay tends to be so long between a doctor ordering something for your loved one and the time it is accomplished. But if your loved one is suffering, or their body is suffering even if they're not conscious to know it,[57] you have a valid reason to become a very squeaky wheel.

Testing and Surgical Delays

There are hundreds of patients in hospitals. If what's been scheduled for the morning doesn't happen by lunchtime, become the squeaky wheel before that day gets longer.

Doctors Round in the Early Morning—Be There

You must be at your loved one's bedside when the doctors round. This cannot be overstated.

Most doctors round between 6:30 to 9 a.m., before their office hours. You must be at your loved one's bedside during those hours (not downstairs in the cafeteria or en route back upstairs, coffee in hand). Be in the room, waiting to consult with the doctors personally. This means you have to get up early enough, every day, to get out of wherever you're staying, eat, enjoy the rush-hour drive through some area you don't know well, find a parking space somewhere in the hospital's orbit, get your coffee, and navigate the hospital labyrinth to your loved one's room by 6:30 a.m., just in case the doc arrives that early. Doctors will not wait for you; they have many patients to see before their first office appointment.

Rounding hours of 6:30 to 9 a.m. are general. Docs can round at any time. Query each and every doctor attending to your loved one to learn exactly when they round.

If you miss the rounds, your alternative is leaving a phone message for each doctor on the case to return your call sometime later in the day. Good luck. Plus, this introduces an unwelcome additional factor: you will no longer be up-to-date on your loved one's condition, which you must monitor constantly.[58]

Um, Where's The Doctor?

One aspect of doctor's scheduling has to do with whether or not a given doctor is rounding at all during the weeks your family inhabits the hospital. This has nothing to do with hospital time and everything to do with who's minding the store.

In my dad's case, he went to the hospital independently to undergo eligibility testing for a coronary pacemaker. His personal physician was the admitting doctor, and she made rounds for some days after his admission, both before and after his condition changed from normal to debilitated. My sister met her during that time. By the time I arrived, she was no longer visiting. My understanding was that she was on vacation.

Doctors often work in teams and stand in for one another. Typically, this occurs within a shared practice. If your doctor's partners are as good as s/he is, you can benefit. If they're not, you've got another instance of discontinuous care.

It turned out that Dad's doc was not on vacation; she was *off rotation*. She was not rounding for several weeks; her partners were. In Dad's case, it developed into a particularly egregious issue.

Ask your loved one's admitting doctor if s/he will be rounding for the expected duration of your loved one's hospitalization and whether any absences during your stay are planned. If your loved one is dying, time is tight, and you have legal business to accomplish, ask the lawyer a similar question: who will be available to help you if the lawyer is in conference or court?[59]

Calendar Considerations

Thursday is the most important day in the hospital. Why? Because the next day is Friday. If something hasn't been ordered by a doctor and Friday dawns, there's a risk that it won't happen until Monday.

Hospitals are much like any other large office, except instead of emptying completely on weekends, they are staffed less and slow down. If you can avoid it, you and your loved one do not want to endure a weekend during which nothing happens except that you all languish while hospital bills rack up.

In addition to scheduling, another issue is who's left to work in the hospital. Most senior personnel will have holidays and weekends off. Most of those working are junior staff.

July is the month when freshly minted interns begin their new jobs; be especially wary of this at teaching hospitals. If possible, schedule elective surgery during other months.

Hospital pharmacies are subject to the same weekend and holiday staffing issues as the hospital itself. This can account for delays in prescriptions being filled during those times.

I'm not suggesting that nothing productive occurs in the hospital during these times, just that the likelihood of delays increases.

Nor am I suggesting that you accept anything less than treatment services, competently provided, with the right supplies and pharmaceuticals for your loved one. There is no reason or excuse for any other treatment.

Who Is That Administering to Your Loved One?

WHO'S POKING OR OTHERWISE MANIPULATING YOUR LOVED ONE? Unless workers are clearly tagged, you may not know the skill level and training of whoever is doing what to your loved one. Staff ranging from registered nurses to technicians may conduct routine procedures. Technicians may have been trained for as little as two weeks in order to perform a single task. This is quite distinct from the multi-year commitment that nursing school represents and a nurse's sensitivity to patient condition.

Below is a typical hierarchical structure for nursing personnel from the bottom up:

Nursing Staff

- Technician: narrowly trained and responsible for certain narrowly defined tasks
- Nurse's Aide (Certified Nursing Assistant/CNA): responsible for taking vital signs, providing personal assistance, and maintaining hygiene
- Licensed Practical Nurse or Licensed Vocational Nurse (LPN or LVN): allowed to administer medications by mouth
- Registered Nurse (RN): has full responsibility for the patient, including starting intravenous drips (IVs), administering IV medications and antibiotics, making patient assessments, reporting to and alerting doctors

The nursing providers listed above are licensed for a scope of practice. Each successively higher level can engage in all the activities that lower levels can, plus the activities at their tier. The particulars of each level may vary from state to state. Investigate at the beginning of each hospitalization to get clear about what treatments each nursing level is authorized to provide. I'd ask the charge nurse for the unit your loved one is in.

Nursing Management

Some nurse managers administer to patients, the upper levels administer at the level of the institution. The only nurse manager you're likely to encounter is a charge nurse, unless a grave ethical crisis was to emerge (in which case, some or even all of the other management-level nurses would attend a treatment group conference along with your patient-family, ethical personnel, and perhaps a lawyer or two).

- Charge Nurse: oversees the nursing floor for a given shift, coordinating patient/nurse staffing needs within a given unit
- Nursing Administrator: responsible for the entire hospital, makes patient admission assignments
- Clinical Manager: manages the budget, personnel levels, and discipline for a given unit
- Department Director: the department administrator
- Director of Nursing: oversees all of the above.

Who is Cutting and Sewing?

The question of who is attending to your loved one extends into surgery, too. Before you thank the surgeon for those nice, neat stitches, you might want to know who exactly stitched the body closed after the main surgical procedure—it may have been an intern. Or perhaps an intern performed part of the surgery itself, under the hopefully watchful eye of the surgeon you've hired on the basis of his or her reputation for positive surgical outcomes.

Before surgery, you may also want to inquire who will be in the operating room during the procedure. You may be surprised to discover that if the procedure requires an implant, a representative of the company making the device will be scrubbed and present in an advisory role. Having an implant manufacturer's expertise at the surgeon's elbow is not bad, it's just one more thing we're not told about.

In general, the more important question would be who else your surgeon plans to allow to operate and their qualifications. Especially given the risks and difficulties associated with curative treatment near end of life, you might want to ensure that only seasoned practitioners will conduct any invasive procedures.

Aside from ED docs, most doctors are independent of hospitals. They make business arrangements for the right to practice at one or more hospitals in their communities (doctors practicing at a hospital are said to have *privileges* there). In previous times, "residents" were exactly that; they lived and worked at the hospital. To some extent, those days are returning, with the advent of the "hospitalist," a doctor in the employ of the hospital. Be sure to ask which doctors are hospitalists and which are independent. On one hand, when a doctor is needed immediately, having hospitalists in-house can be useful. On the other hand, adding hospitalists to the treatment group may add to discontinuity of care, where a variety of specialists without an authoritative leader each attend to less than the full patient. Hospitalists work on shifts, thus information about your loved one's condition requires handing off several times per day.

Hospitals are Multiracial Environments

As with other segments of our society, there exists a racial/ethnic divide in hospitals. Two, actually.

As a white man, I have experience with only one of them. The one I don't have experience with deserves mention. People of color share a concern that the system devalues their lives compared to the lives of white people. This concern arises near and during end of life, when some people of color question whether or not the system provides as much care as it seems to for whites. I'm not qualified to comment on this, but I mention it here to acknowledge an important issue of which I discuss related aspects in chapter 9, "The Option to Die in PEACE."

The second divide I am familiar with. Depending upon where you live, where you're hospitalized, your financial status, and your family's ethnicity, you may find yourself in a novel environment. In our experiences, most of the people who float in and out of hospital rooms are not doctors, nurses, or even technicians. The docs round once daily in the early morning and may occasionally appear at other times. Nurses don't come by just to check in on your loved one; nurses round on a schedule related to administering fluids, medications, and other treatments. In the interim, patients are left entirely alone (although this is the exact opposite of Mom-and-Apple-Pie Care, during which extended periods of quiet are a signal to the caregiver to engage in a quick patient check).

Except for those who arrive to set up specialized equipment, everyone else is more or less involved with hospitality services: food delivery and removal; supply delivery; cleaning; bathing and repositioning the patient. These are low-paying jobs. In many areas of the country, they are staffed by the most recent immigrant groups and others on the lower socio-economic scale in the community.

The hospital room is a place where the most intimate care is provided to a virtually naked loved one—an unshowered, unshampooed, unshaven, unkempt, weakened, pain-ridden person who just a few days before inhabited his or her own home. You and your family are hanging out there in various stages of stress, worry, fatigue, and with whatever emotional baggage you bring together. No matter your ethnicity or color, chances are good that some number among the staff assisting your loved one in intimate bedside ways, including those sent by the nursing company you hire to assist, will be of a different ethnic or racial origin than your family. This was the case in Dad's hospitalization.

Despite what value we may receive from our multiracial society, we may not have close personal relationships outside our own ethnic or racial groups. The hospital room, during very vulnerable times, may end up being a first opportunity.

I value diversity in America. I'm white; my personal physician happens to be black. I don't understand countries where inhabitants insist on uniformity, let alone want it badly enough to commit atrocities to obtain it.

I think eradicating cultural bias is a good thing. Doing so at this time and place may add an unexpected element of surprise and stress to an already complex situation. The good news is that if you're open to tenderness, the few degrees of heat this may add to the crucible will warm your heart in the long run.

Firing Nurses, Doctors, and Hospitals

FIRING TREATMENT PROVIDERS IS AN EXTREME ACTION.

You may consider me testy for using the term "firing." Consider the four firing anecdotes below and decide for yourself how you would have felt in these circumstances.

We removed one technician and two nurses during Dad's hospitalization. Had we had our wits about us during Mom's hospitalization, we would have fired the institution and had her moved to one that actually manifested care (rather than denying their failure to) and offered family care rather than family exclusion.

Hospital patients have explicit rights. Know them: read the patient rights brochure and lobby placard.

A Technician Fired

Before I arrived on the scene, Judy fired a technician who caused unnecessary pain and risk of infection during a routine blood draw:

> EARLY ONE MORNING, A TECHNICIAN CAME to draw blood from Mort's inner forearm. Although his left arm was not the afflicted one, the skin was somewhat delicate. Due to his heart condition, he was on blood thinners and thus was more prone to bleeding.
>
> A square of tape was in place on Mort's arm from a previous draw. The tech just ripped it off, peeling some skin with it. The area started to bleed. In that instant, the risk of a new infection site was created.

Judy, who had been sitting at the bedside, jumped up and exclaimed, "What the hell are you doing?" She then told the tech to get out, not come back, and to send someone else to draw the blood.

Nurse One Fired

The first nurse to go was so shockingly rude and damaging that we failed to respond immediately because we were stunned by his behavior. My sister, who had fired the technician the week before, was doubly stunned that Dad was being subjected to a second instance of careless treatment during his hospitalization.

> TO HELP STAFF WORK WITH DAD'S INFIRMITIES, we hung signs made in large, bold lettering over his bed. We were advised by the nurses that hanging signs directly over the bed is a preferred method to communicate vital information about a patient.

Providers (including staff) know to look for and familiarize themselves with these short messages. We posted two:

DO NOT TOUCH MORT'S INFLAMED,
PAINFUL RIGHT WRIST

MORT CAN HEAR AND COMMUNICATE PERFECTLY
WHEN YOU SPEAK SLOWLY AND CLEARLY
NEAR HIS RIGHT EAR

In trots a guy we've never seen in the week we've been there. Chattering away, he doesn't so much as greet my very awake father, look for (let alone at) the signs, identify himself, say hello to Judy and I, or inquire about anything. Rather, seeing the IV drips attached to Dad's left hand, he makes a direct beeline for Dad's inflamed and painful right wrist. Dad, a guy who never showed he was in pain, began roaring even before this nurse made contact, which he did anyway, squeezing Dad's wrist in an attempt to get a pulse.

I should have ushered the nurse out of the room right then. Instead, we advised him about Dad's condition and the content of the signs. This made no positive impression on him; he retorted that he knew how to do his job and that he was a professional. We told him to leave.

I left Judy and Dad in the room, marched to the nursing station, and engaged the charge nurse. I asked who the guy was, described his actions, and ordered that he be immediately removed from my father's care and never step foot in Dad's room again. She nodded knowingly, and that was the last we saw of him.

The lesson here is stark: if you see mistreatment by any staff member, stop that person *immediately*. Do not let them continue *any* patient contact. Accompany them away, then go immediately to the nursing station to report the mistreatment and resolve the issue.

Nurse Two Fired

The second nurse we fired was the hospice intake nurse.

Being admitted into hospice is a profound passage. It demands compassion and exactitude. It is, as we experienced it, a well-thought out, unhurried procedure. Communication is precise, and redundant. They want to make sure that you know what hospice is, isn't, and that you're admitting yourself voluntarily. Mental clarity must be demonstrated by the principal and/or personal representative during a family interview. Various legal forms must be signed. Intake is conducted by an experienced intake nurse.

THIS PARTICULAR NURSE *was personable and seemed professional. During the latter stages of the intake, after Judy and I had left for several hours, it became clear that some of the information he had imparted to the family was in error.*

I know that people are only human, but the last place and time you want erroneous information is during the intake of your second parent into a hospice on a Friday afternoon.

In two instances the errors were small and we endured their consequences. A third error was egregious—a direct misrepresentation of either my father's state, wishes, or the family's orientation (I no longer remember the details) by the intake nurse to Dad's admitting physician.

Previously this nurse had misinformed only the family; this time he misinformed the key provider. In so doing, he broke any trust we had in him. That this occurred on the brink of moving Dad to hospice was intolerable.

As soon as I resolved the error I marched, this time to the hospice wing, where I asked for the social worker in charge of my father's case. I was profoundly disturbed and requested we meet privately. (As did every provider in the hospital, she would have unquestioningly proceeded with the conversation in the middle of the hallway.)

Behind the closed door of her tiny office, I recounted the three errors and told her, "This man will not utter one more syllable to any member of our family. I want him off the case and for him to stay completely away from all of us for the duration of my father's hospice stay." She agreed, and it was done.

The Hospital We Should Have Fired

I mentioned earlier about how the worst, anti-family ICUs greatly restrict family visitation, even to the point of banning family and personal representatives during the only hours doctors habitually round.

Such was the case where my mother was bedridden. This place was a disaster. Orderlies banged storage closet doors in the unit, showing a profound lack of respect for patients and family members.

The unit was kept locked. All the patients' family members herded at those locked doors each morning at 11 a.m. ("opening time"). The late hour notwithstanding, we were usually kept waiting for unknown reasons. It seemed like the slightest medical snafu with any patient would cause staff to re-lock the unit and chase all families away, banished to queue at those damn double doors again. The unit was locked at each shift change ("report," it's called, when the outgoing shift reports to the incoming shift). For efficiency? Respite? Privacy? Secrecy? Who knows?

Family members were either highly discouraged or actively prohibited from engaging in patient comfort—even professionally competent people like my sister. My mother's greatly lowered internal temperature (a profound medical problem) was ignored.

One of my first interviewees was a former hospital nurse who'd gone into private practice. A year after her own mother's passing, she was still in massive distress about their family's mistreatment. Imagine our joint shock when it surfaced that her mother had been hospitalized and died in the very same ICU my mother had.

Both of these veteran nurses, my sister and this woman, had been rendered impotent and reduced to tears by the treatment they endured in this unit.

We should have fired the hospital. The procedure, as I understand it, is to advise the admitting physician of your dissatisfaction and your intention to leave. Ask the admitting physician what other nearby facilities s/he has visitation privileges at and for their recommendation for a replacement hospital with the desired attributes. That hospital must be willing and able to accept the patient. An additional potential burden may be whether or not your loved one's insurance company places limits on which hospitals may be used (assuming private insurance is in effect).

You still have your notebook and are taking extensive notes, documenting everything, right? Because you'll also need to see if you have an insurance fight on your hands (unless you resign to paying the thousand dollars or more it'll cost to move a very infirm patient from one ICU to another across town). Since I have no experience doing this, I have no other input, except to say that patients cannot be forced to stay in any institution against their will (or against yours as their Medical Power of Attorney) as long as there's another institution that agrees to admit them.

Hospitalization Experienced as a Crucible

A CRUCIBLE IS A PLACE OR SITUATION IN WHICH WE ARE SUBJECT to intense forces that directly challenge us. The concentration of forces during hospitalizations, especially terminal ones, is profound. These forces press against us. They appear as competing interests, including the medical, ethical, moral, spiritual, religious, financial, and legal. They invoke the core of our humanity. These interests overlap in an unfamiliar environment, a compressed time frame, and with the highest stakes...stakes so high no one wants to openly discuss them.

Under these conditions, the emotional impact of accumulated extrinsic shocks is amplified. We figuratively, and perhaps literally, recoil. We experience each extrinsic shock like an improvised explosive device (IED).[60] Our equilibrium gets blasted, and along with it our decision-making capacity.

From boredom and helplessness to confusion, fear, shock, agony, and grief, few institutional experiences arouse more challenging emotions than a hospitalization. Few situations demand so much of us to resolve. Few situations affect us as profoundly as a terminal hospitalization that we feel, in our gut, is wrong in its very context (due to the very nature of a hospital as a place in which to experience one's final days).

And it gets worse if we lose already diminishing opportunities to commune with our loved one and to receive direction about their wishes. Aside from our loved one's recovery, these two opportunities represent our most vital interests during hospitalizations. If infringed upon, they cannot be recovered; they have been stolen, further deepening the emotional impact.

Each lost opportunity for communion and communication is vital. It takes enormous bravery to acknowledge imminent death, especially between a parent and adult child. We may not get it said on the first or second try. We need all possible opportunities—without infringement—to commune and receive direction, because we may use many of them in false starts, or let them pass without utilizing them due to ignorance.

Lost opportunities to commune with one another during the end days can haunt survivors for years. They carry seeds of regret, which tend to sprout. Without direction from the patient, our loved one, the burden of making life-and-death choices will fall to us, their personal representative. Long after decisions are made to end treatment, the burden around having made them, and having *had* to make them, can pulse with a life of its own among the survivors who have taken this responsibility.

If All Else Fails

What if you learn the lessons in *Notes from the Waiting Room* too late to apply them? What if your loved one insisting on hospitalized dying? What if your experience of their dying is worse than you feel it could have been? What then? What can we do in the face of helplessness, of acknowledging personal shortcomings that we feel may have contributed to complicating a loved one's death...or of making it less peaceful? If your loved one has already died under these conditions, what now?

Be kind to yourself. Assuming that you did what you were able to do (even if that was less than you might have been capable of doing), take yourself off the hook. You may have been part of the situation (a case of shared responsibility), but in all likelihood you weren't the lone decider. It may take some time, soul-searching, and parsing, but you will likely conclude that a great many forces were colliding and numerous issues were playing out during your patient-family's stay in the crucible (and the balance of this book may help you in that process).

Allow yourself to recover through whatever means arise in your life. In my case, prior to my parents' deaths I never napped. Shortly after Dad's death, the emotional weight I felt pressed me earthward. I began napping: on the living room floor, the couch, the hammock, the outdoor recliner, the indoor recliner, the chair I use at lakesides during windsurfing sessions. What would account for a sudden need to nap so frequently? I concluded that my soul was fatigued.

I suspect that some large number of us do not get many chances to master a time of life made so complex that it's become a crucible. Even after experiencing one death, each other death proceeds differently; every death can take us by surprise.

Help others learn what you learn. Help your remaining family members, friends, and perhaps acquaintances if the circumstances allow.

Accept dying and death. In my case, although the circumstances were less than optimal, it was not a bad thing that my father died when he did. Learn to see the end days in a new way. I propose a way to accept dying and death in this book's last section, "The Imperative to Change End of Life."

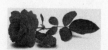

Who's Where, When, Why, for How Long, and Other Turns through the Hospital Maze Recap: What You Can Do

If your loved one is hospitalized, document everything throughout each day and night. Maintain notes (your personal "chart") or keep a journal.

Be an effective question-asker! *Start now.* Has this chapter answered all your questions about:

- What constitutes hospital time and how it "flows"?
- When and where to make face-to-face contact with physicians?
- The importance of certain days of the week in the hospital?
- The range of people treating and assisting your loved one and the management hierarchy above them?
- The occasional need to fire providers or hospitals and how to go about doing so?

- Beginning steps to take to unburden yourself regarding a loved one's death?

If you do not have all the information you need, write your questions down. How will you get them answered? Reread this chapter? Internet research? Library research? Consulting with family and friends? A phone call to a professional or organization? Go online or pick up the phone book, find a likely contact, and send the email or place the call.

7 | The Complete Do-Not-Resuscitate Conversation

EXTRINSIC SHOCK ONE: "SHE'S NOT A DNR!"
Mom is intubated in the ICU, unconscious, unresponsive, and possibly comatose. Dad, Judy, and I are there with her admitting doctor, who happens to be both of my parents' cardiologist.

A week earlier, complaining of fatigue and possessing congenitally unhealthy cholesterol levels despite rigorous adherence to a low-fat diet, she had gone to the outpatient clinic for evaluation of a heart arrhythmia.

We were told that while waiting under observation, Mom experienced difficulty breathing. No family member was with her at the time, and I do not know the nature of her difficulty. She accepted breathing support, although we don't know whether that was a mask or full intubation. All we know is that she wound up in the ICU, unconscious, on mechanical ventilation, a breathing tube down her trachea.

Her cardiologist discussed the treatment plan with the family members. We hoped to be able to restore her equilibrium (by elevating her internal temperature), remove the breathing tube ("extubation"), and see if she could breathe on her own.

Either Judy or I inquired about the relationship between her Do-Not-Resuscitate (DNR) status and the treatment plan. The doc replied that she was not a DNR (a patient with a DNR status becomes "a DNR"). I happened to be watching Dad as he heard this statement. His body involuntarily recoiled; he took this news in as if he'd been speared.

Let's put this in context. The family had conducted advance planning and had executed the appropriate papers. Both elders had their wits about them and, as business managers in their working years, were used to keeping their papers in order. One might presume their cardiologist, with whom they'd had a long-standing and active relationship, would know their DNR status and wishes. I have no idea if Mom's paperwork was submitted upon admission. In any case, Dad was under the impression that her DNR status was known and in effect. Apparently, the staff did not have paperwork indicating her DNR status. We did not know that they didn't have her status correctly charted because there was no discussion with us about it. As family, we suffered the consequences of this lack of discussion and forecasting.

Picture an eighty-three-year-old man standing over his spouse of sixty years lying intubated in the ICU. He was not expecting this situation. Everyone, himself included, thought he would die first due to various ailments, primary among them heart disease.

Despite his robust intelligence, he stands there in a state of shock. The doc says his wife, who ought to be DNR status, is not.

It was a needless jolt that had real consequences. It took us almost half a day to drive home to the neighboring town, obtain the original DNR paper, return to the hospital, and get a copy to the ICU nursing staff. DNR submitted and in effect, right? No. It took another day for the doctor to return, put the order into Mom's chart, for the chart to return to the nurses' station, and for the nurses to flag the chart. Had Mom's heart *stopped during this time, they would have been legally bound to call Code Blue and have the resuscitation team swarm down upon her. When a patient "codes" (as suffering heart or respiratory failure is referred to), the family is kicked out. In some ICUs, during codes they close the unit to all of the other patients' visitors, too.*

EXTRINSIC SHOCK TWO: "SHE'S A DNR!"
It is now a few days later, and the various signs by which we interpret Mom's condition continue to slowly improve. More oxygen is in her blood. Her blood pressure is up a little. The amount of air being mechanically forced into her lungs has been lowered, i.e., her autonomic breathing has slightly improved.

The docs are ready to try to extubate her.

This is a make-or-break process. She will breathe on her own or she will not; she will prove viable, else we'll have to come to grips with letting her go. We're about twelve days into her ICU stay, and that duration is not a good sign.

It's a replay of the earlier scene: the family and the cardiologist discussing Mom's condition and the treatment plan, except that Mom's DNR has been charted and she's now no-code status, "a DNR" in the vernacular. Suddenly a thought occurs to me, and I question the doc: "What happens if she can't breathe when you extubate her? Will you shove the tube back in?"

The doc looks at me as if I were an alien. "Of course not," he says, "she's a DNR!"

The room went silent except for the hissing of Mom's ventilator. I looked at Dad. He was stricken.

Neither he nor my sister had thought to ask the question I had just asked. Unfortunately, this cardiologist's bedside manner did not include briefing the family on a range of possible outcomes. Nor had he introduced the topic of physician interpretation of clinical responsibilities and choices at the *intersection of a patient's resuscitation status and treatment.*

It was too much. Here we were, on the precipice of a procedure from which there was no turning back now that Mom's DNR status was in effect. My father was not ready for the specter of his lifelong partner dying that afternoon. He postponed pulling out the tube feeding oxygen to Mom's lungs. This, of course, meant that she would languish another day or more in intensive care. And although we were not thinking in financial terms at the time, those additional days would add to the national cost of the last few weeks of life.

FOR THOSE IN ACUTE NEED OR CRISIS

RESUSCITATION DOES NOT LEND ITSELF TO SUMMARIZA-
TION. It is a complex topic with intense moral, emotional, medical, and legal ramifications. The best I can
say to those with little time to lose is to do these things
in rapid succession: (1) find out what your loved one's
resuscitation desires are and (2) find out if their hospital status matches their desire. Visually check your
loved one's hospital chart at the nursing station; any
Do-Not-Resuscitate (DNR) status must appear <u>in</u> and be
flagged <u>on</u> the chart by a doctor's order, or it is not in
effect.

Without resuscitation, anyone who arrests (stops
breathing or whose heart stops) will die then and there.
With resuscitation, in general, we have a very slight
chance of partial recovery (leaving us disabled), and a
scant chance of full recovery. Real life is not like TV
hospital shows.

Resuscitation attempts are virtually impossible to
stop once begun. They continue unabated for 45-60 minutes. At their fullest, they are invasive, messy procedures that may appear to be assaults (which they are if
resuscitation is not desired).

Unlike defibrillators used to resuscitate those whose hearts have stopped, BREATHING TUBES HAVE MORE THAN ONE USE. Lay people think of intubation as a resuscitation technology. Doctors view it in three ways: (1) resuscitation in emergencies, (2) standard operating procedure during surgeries, and (3) treatment at other times. This surprising fact turns the intersection of patient autonomy and treatment goals into potential quagmires -- ETHICAL GRAY ZONES. Do not expect to be advised about these in advance. Plan to pose questions prior to any procedure during which resuscitation is or could be an issue.

ASK EVERY ATTENDING DOCTOR TO EXPLAIN THEIR INTERPRETATION OF THEIR RESPONSIBILITY REGARDING YOUR LOVED ONE'S DNR STATUS. You may be surprised to hear different answers depending upon the doctor and the environment. Be prepared to revisit these queries if and as your loved one's condition deteriorates. Options exist, yet must be unearthed -- so ask. Unless a doctor needs a decision from you at this moment, you've got time to read this chapter and engage in the conversations you ought to have with (in this order) your loved one, your family, your loved one's admitting physician, and the rest of the treatment group.

The Complete Do-Not-Resuscitate Conversation

THE SPECTER OF YOUR LOVED ONE DOWN AND OUT during a serious or terminal hospitalization is more than enough to cope with. Adding extrinsic shocks on top of it is unconscionable. In my experience, the most disruptive extrinsic shocks were related to resuscitation.

In the absence of adequate forecasting about the many issues bearing on whether or not to resuscitate, extrinsic shocks around resuscitation are a given. I think it safe to say that you are bound to encounter them, since heroic resuscitation is the medical default mode, if not the public expectation (*we* are part of the system), during medical crises.

The typical resuscitation conversation might go like this: "If you don't want to be resuscitated, say so in an advance directive document" (I don't recall hearing more from the media during the days of Terri Schiavo's ultimate demise). The reality is that such a "conversation" is terribly and overly simplistic. Real life is *far* more complex.

Resuscitation is a serious event medically, ethically, emotionally, and legally. You would think that a thorough and detailed conversation would be *required* as a matter of policy. Let's have that conversation now—a sober and far-ranging conversation. Let's illuminate the many aspects of, and gray areas around, resuscitation.

> **WARNING: Submitting a Do-Not-Resuscitate directive to the hospital (assuming you have one) is the tip of the iceberg. Submission alone does not cause DNR status to take effect. Even after DNR status is in effect, unless you have discussions with each physician attending to your loved one, you will not know how each doctor interprets an effective DNR and their responsibility in relation to it as treatment unfolds.**

ALTHOUGH NO LAW REQUIRES you to have executed advance directives,[61] actions regarding resuscitation ought to begin during hospital admission. If you have a Living Will and/or a DNR form, admission is the time to submit them. (The clerk should make copies; be SURE to keep the originals yourself.) The suite of forms includes the Living Will, Medical Power of Attorney, HIPAA authorization and release and, if desired, a Do-Not-Resuscitate (DNR) form (assuming the patient's physician has already filled one out). For people submitting a DNR form, it is an extremely important document. You may assume that the act of submitting it means that it is in effect. *You may be wrong.*

Early in 2005 the Do-Not-Resuscitate order, or DNR, became part of the United States' national vocabulary due to the extraordinary circumstances surrounding the final removal of feeding tubes from Terri Schiavo, a woman maintained in a persistent vegetative state for fifteen years.[62]

Unfortunately, the national conversation was a short one consisting of only one pragmatic fact: if you do not want to be resuscitated, say so in an advance directive.

This was and remains a simplistic, inadequate DNR conversation. If you do no more, you leave yourself open to treatment you may not desire, and of having your family's emotional rug pulled out from under them in many ways.

The complete in-hospital DNR conversation involves the following questions:

- What is resuscitation?
- What's a DNR directive?
- What's a DNR form?
- What's the difference between a DNR form and a Living Will?
- What is required for a DNR to take effect in the hospital?
- How long does it take for a DNR to take effect in the hospital?
- How do you verify that a DNR is in effect in the hospital?
- What happens if a DNR order is not in effect?
- What happens, or doesn't happen, when a DNR is in effect?
- Are all DNRs the same?
- What if the doctor will not recognize a DNR that has been properly filed and should be in effect?
- Are DNRs permanent?
- What about DNRs for events outside the hospital?
- How effective are resuscitation attempts?
- What are the ethical gray zones governing the application of DNRs under various circumstances?

- How does each provider view and feel about patient resuscitation directives? Under what conditions would s/he engage in resuscitation or withhold it? Might these conditions arise during any treatment provided your loved one? If so, how will the provider behave should treatment goals and a resuscitation directive collide?
- When is the application of resuscitation technology considered routine treatment rather than life support?
- Will new resuscitation techniques change how we approach our resuscitation directives?

Note that this conversation does not include any examination of the moral issues about whether to resuscitate or not. That deeply personal decision is every person's alone. We'll discuss contemplating that sort of decision in chapter 9, "The Option to Die in PEACE."

Resuscitation and its Relationship with Treatment Goals

PERHAPS THE MOST IMPORTANT ASPECT TO UNDERSTAND about resuscitation is that the professionals who provide it do so under legal constraints, moral requirements, and ethical assumptions.

The legal constraint is simple: in the absence of legally acceptable and instantly recognizable instructions to withhold resuscitation, providers assisting an affected person will resuscitate. This is true inside the hospital, the home, or on the street.

The moral requirement for providers to resuscitate is that when they *can* save a life, they *must* save a life. Doing so is why they became healthcare providers or first responders.[63]

The ethical aspect of resuscitation is not so well known: a predominant medical stance is that for anyone undergoing curative treatment, resuscitation is, by default, an acceptable, even necessary part of that treatment.

The relationship between treatment goals and resuscitation was first introduced to me by an emergency department physician whom I'll call Dr. D. I initially queried Dr. D about the finer points of applied DNR orders. I queried him primarily because of the shocking moments my family and I experienced regarding DNRs in each of my parents' cases. The first two moments were related; I described them in this chapter's opening. The shocks arose due to lack of forecasting and questionable procedural protocol. A third, unexpected incident involved what we perceived as very fine ethical slicing and dicing, resulting in our moving my father from curative care to hospice—a one-way ticket in his case. Like the first two, this situation also arose with no forewarning.

Further, the issue of resuscitation is in most of our futures, especially for anyone hospitalized at or near end of life.

Dr. D suggested that more important than focusing on DNRs was to understand and focus on treatment goals. He said where there's hope, there's a treatment plan. Dr. D suggested that:

- DNR considerations are subservient to active treatment (in other words, we ought to focus less on resuscitation issues and more on the goals and course of treatment).

- Active treatment ought to include a thorough, up-front discussion of treatment risks and benefits, including potential complications (i.e., forecasting).

- Treatment goals are subject to change.

- The introduction, use, and removal of life support ought to be based on current treatment goals.

- DNRs are not inconsistent with active curative treatment. A DNR order ought *not* be misconstrued by practitioners as an order to abandon active treatment, provide only comfort care (palliate), or prepare for the patient's death.

- Putting a patient in intensive care and applying life support is not necessarily out of the question for someone who is a DNR.

- Physicians define their responsibilities regarding DNRs in different ways. For patients who arrest during a physician-initiated procedure, doctors could honor the DNR and let the patient die without resuscitation. Or, on the grounds that their intervention caused the arrest, they could resuscitate to try to restore the patient to their earlier state, then consult the family.

Dr. D's milieu is the emergency room, where there can be literally no time to ponder resuscitation issues. These issues, however, relate to the hospitalization of any person, especially those near or in a terminal condition (which includes most of our elderly...interpreting what constitutes a terminal condition is, of course, a moving target subject to social, religious, and ethical values). By emphasizing treatment goals, Dr. D is helpful in providing the context to examine resuscitation issues. After all, we go to hospitals to try to solve acute medical problems, go home, and keep on living.

Beginning our resuscitation conversation by acknowledging the importance of treatment goals expands our thinking regarding DNRs. But doing so does not change the fact that DNR complexities exist, treatment goals notwithstanding, particularly in the absence of forecasting. Patient-families deserve to have a complete range of possibilities to contemplate. People need time to prepare to make decisions in advance of having to actually specify or enforce a resuscitation directive. Because— it bears restating—effectively managing resuscitation goes far beyond stating wishes in advance directives.

Practicalities and Legalities of Resuscitation

What is Resuscitation?

Resuscitation is the application of potentially life-saving procedures including:

- Restarting the heart by physical, mechanical, or chemical means, i.e. cardiopulmonary resuscitation (CPR) defibrillation,[64] or injection
- Applying an invasive[65] mechanized breathing apparatus administering oxygen, or "ventilating," by inserting a large tube down the throat and windpipe (referred to as *intubation*).

What's a DNR Directive? What's a DNR Form?
What's a DNR Order?

Patients make directives; doctors issue treatment orders. You and I and our loved ones can issue a personal *DNR statement or directive*. The statement is one of several made in an advance directive form (Living Will). When the form is signed, the statement is intended to prohibit the application of potentially life-saving resuscitation measures under certain conditions.

A *DNR form* is filled out by a physician after discussion with his or her patient—and perhaps the patient's spouse, adult children, and Medical Power of Attorney—if the DNR is being created during hospitalization or while the patient is incapacitated. DNR forms may also be filled out by physicians for patients when their condition brings them closer to, rather than further from, dying of some medical complication.

A *DNR order* is a doctor addition to a patient's hospital chart officially notifying hospital staff of the patient's DNR status.

These are the basic differences between DNR directives, forms, and orders (although more details exist, which I cover below). The more important aspect is what these differences mean under various resuscitation scenarios.

What's the Difference Between a Living Will and a DNR Form?

A Living Will sets forth a range of possible conditions and the treatments you want or do not want under those conditions. It provides guidance. Although intended to be legally binding, it must be known and seen by responders immediately in a crisis situation before they begin resuscitation.

A DNR form, once signed by a doctor, is an official medical mandate for the person named on the form not to be resuscitated. The form may be a paper of a certain color designated by a state (and, in some states, only original documents of that color are valid). The DNR form may take the "form" of a bracelet issued by a state. In either case, it must be seen by first responders immediately in a crisis situation, or else they will begin resuscitation. Should they see it, they are legally (and ethically) relieved from resuscitating the person named on the form.

Living Wills take many forms and run multiple pages. A Living Will must be read through and its DNR directive located. By contrast, an official DNR form or bracelet can be instantly *seen, understood, and validated* by first responders.

What is Required for a DNR to Take Effect in the Hospital?

The act of submitting a DNR directive or form to a hospital admissions clerk does not make it effective. In the hospital setting, only these related actions make a DNR effective: (1) the clerk must pass along a copy of the form to be included in the patient's chart, (2) a doctor must write an order verifying that the DNR status be put into effect, (3) that order must be entered directly onto the patient's chart, and (4) the chart must be flagged so that the nurses can instantly notice your loved one's DNR status to prevent your loved one from being mistakenly "coded," resulting in a resuscitation team running to their bedside and commencing resuscitation.

How Long does it Take for a DNR to Take Effect in the Hospital?

The delay in making a DNR effective in the hospital depends upon the links and kinks in the communication chain between you, the administration, the admitting doctor, and the unit nursing staff. The best practice is for you to verify your loved one's DNR status immediately, with admissions, the admitting physician, and the nurse in charge of each unit your loved one ends up bedded in.

How do You Verify that the DNR is in Effect in the Hospital?

To ensure that your loved one's DNR is actually in effect, you must look and see with your own eyes that 1) the doctor's order exists on your loved one's chart, and 2) whatever system the nursing staff uses to flag that chart (and thus the patient) as "a DNR" has been implemented.

Double check at every stage beginning with admission. Make sure admission has copied the DNR form. Make sure the admitting doctor is aware of the form and has entered a DNR order into your loved one's chart. Then, sashay on up to the nursing station and ask how they flag DNR patient charts. Ask to see your loved one's chart and, specifically, the doctor's order and the nurse's DNR designation. It'll be some visual cue, affixed in some manner so as to be visible at a moment's notice, perhaps a red sticker on the spine of a three-ring binder. Assess the visual cue to satisfy yourself that it is easily visible at a glance and unlikely to get lost or covered.

Is this supplanting nurse oversight? Yes, it is! And it's OK; if you ask pleasantly or matter-of-factly, they'll show you, and your working relationship with the nurses will remain intact. They understand how vitally important these matters are to your patient-family.

What Happens (or Doesn't Happen) When a DNR is in Effect?

With a DNR in effect, no resuscitation efforts will be made or ought to be made, no matter what occurs. Be very clear about one immutable aspect of resuscitation: if someone needs it and refuses it, they will die then and there in a few minutes or less of cardiac or respiratory arrest, whichever brought them down.

What Happens if a DNR is Not in Effect?

If a DNR is *not* in effect, a series of irreversible activities will occur in a reported medical emergency. By "reported" medical emergency, I mean heart or respiratory failure while hospitalized or in the presence of emergency responders who have responded to a 911 call. It's called Full Code, Code Blue, or just Code; occasionally "Core" (in some parts of the country). When a patient "codes," a team of a half-dozen intently focused personnel will swarm upon the patient and initiate potentially rib-cracking chest compressions. If necessary, they'll add other aspects of cardio-pulmonary resuscitation (CPR):

- Defibrillation (electric jolts) to try to jump-start the heart's rhythm
- Introduce mechanical ventilation—intubation by breathing tube, whereby a machine fills the lungs with air
- Attempt to inject rescue medications through a large vein, typically in the groin area (these are not applied like inoculations; the groin may be jabbed repeatedly in a frantic attempt to locate and penetrate the vein)
- Continue these resuscitation activities unabated for 45-60 minutes before stopping and having a doctor pronounce the patient dead.

These people have a single focus, and you cannot stop them. Even if you believe a DNR to be in effect, only a doctor can order a resuscitation stopped after it has started (remember, laws govern EMT responsibilities). You might try showing a DNR directive or form and possibly your legal right to direct the patient's care (Medical Power of Attorney) in order to begin to reverse the state the patient may be in as a result of resuscitation efforts. Assuming the patient hasn't died or recovered, they are now on life support. Removing it is neither a quick or trivial matter.

Real life resuscitation neither plays out nor ends like those shown on television hospital dramas. The act of resuscitation can be messy business. Twenty-some years ago I witnessed my father receiving chest compressions and defibrillation during a heart attack at age sixty-five. Fortunately, his heart stabilized quickly and the resuscitation was "orderly." I have read, however, of resuscitations that get very messy,[66] with naked patients arms and legs akimbo—especially when the efforts continue for the better part of an hour and require a full court press of interventions.

Determining your resuscitation wishes in advance requires clear thinking. Part of the issue is that the way we view resuscitation changes depending upon circumstances. What appears unwarranted in one context might seem desirable in another. A helpful resource when considering resuscitation directives is the work of Linda Emanuel. Emanuel postulated various scenarios and asked patients to consider whether or not they would want resuscitation in each instance. Apparently Emanuel's work was considered ground-breaking, although on reading the scenarios, years after my own experiences, I found them to lack the kind of nuance that real life is likely to contain.[67]

For the very elderly and/or infirm, resuscitation may be part of what's known as the heroic pathway. My understanding of "heroic pathway" is that it begins where the medical prognosis turns negative—that is, the patient in all likelihood will not survive. I'm not suggesting we arbitrarily dismiss resuscitation, but do be clear about what it is and under which conditions it ought to be performed. My dad's resuscitation and subsequent cardiac double-bypass operation at age sixty-five added almost twenty years to his life. In contrast, resuscitation at or near end stage in the elderly may cause more bodily and emotional harm than it prevents.

What if Providers Will Not Recognize an In-effect DNR?

If a doctor will not recognize an in-effect DNR and insists on resuscitation, you've got a severe problem. Ideally, the best way to deal with such a problem is to prevent it from occurring at all, by interviewing your loved one's doctors and ascertaining that you and they are in agreement about resuscitation matters in your loved one's case—including the doctors' interpretation of their responsibilities under certain treatment conditions in light of the DNR status.

If resuscitation is begun despite the DNR, you might try yelling that this patient has been charted as a no-code. In such an instance, either a medical mistake or a breach of medical ethics (or both) has occurred.

An instance like this would justify subsequently removing those responsible from the case and insisting that they and the hospital complete their ethical obligation by assisting you in finding replacements who will honor legally recognized directives. Help for dealing with these issues is readily available in many hospitals, as reviewed in the forecasting chapter.

Are DNR Orders Permanent?

As patients, we have the right to accept or refuse treatment. In the context of a DNR conversation, this means that we can rescind (cancel) a DNR decision at any time (make sure it's before you need resuscitation!).

Lesser known is that hospitals *require* us to rescind DNR status during surgery performed under general anesthesia. This is because surgery under general anesthesia requires the use of mechanical ventilation, i.e., the breathing tube, which is part of how a patient is kept alive during surgery. Thus, anyone undergoing surgery under a general must agree to "resuscitation" *during* the surgery, and to the *reintroduction* of resuscitation within some period should cardiac arrest occur post-op. The duration of the rescission varies by hospital; it could end when leaving the post-surgical recovery room or extend up to *forty-eight* hours post-op.

Still lesser known is how individual doctors view their responsibilities to patients when their direct actions intersect with a patient's DNR status (we'll discuss the doctor/DNR intersection shortly).

Are All DNR Forms the Same?

DNR forms are not all the same. I'm aware of four, two used in the hospital and two used outside the hospital. The four options I've seen are:
- A Living Will, which includes a DNR directive, intended for submission upon admission to a hospital. A personal representative,

while ethically bound by the directive, is not legally bound to follow it. Best practice is to keep a copy of a DNR directive in your wallet or purse.

- A hospital's own non-revocable DNR form executed by a patient in the hospital. This form differs from the Living Will in a critical way: It cannot be overridden by a Medical Power of Attorney. If the patient executes this form and subsequently becomes incapacitated (unable to direct her care), no resuscitation will occur. Period. I do not know if all hospitals offer this option.

- A "refrigerator" DNR, a form signed by a doctor and placed on the refrigerator or in the front hall of a home, where, hopefully, first responders to a 911 call will see it and refrain from beginning resuscitation for the person named on the form. If the named person is bedridden, hanging the form from the bed inside of a plastic sleeve is sometimes recommended.

- An official state-issued DNR bracelet or medallion, which requires proof of a doctor-signed DNR form to obtain. Bracelets may be serial numbered.

DNR Status and Emergency Responders

Emergency responders are those that are first on the scene after a call for help. This may be fire or police officers or emergency medical technicians (ambulance personnel) responding to a 911 call. There are three locations where a person could fail and responders would need to know whether or not to resuscitate: home, hospital, or elsewhere (let's call it "the street"). With home and hospital covered (via refrigerator DNR, bracelet, and a doctor's DNR order), the remaining variable is the street.

The impetus for a national emergency telephone number began in the late 1950s to report fires. A decade later its role was expanded to report emergencies of all types, and the telephone system eventually assigned 911 for that purpose. By the turn of the century, the use of 911 on a nationwide basis was codified in law. Somewhere along the way, making a 911 call came to be construed as implied consent to cardiopulmonary resuscitation (CPR). This means that responders to a 911 call assume that resuscitation has been consented to by, or on behalf of, the person to whom they are providing emergency treatment. If the patient is incapacitated responders will resuscitate on the assumption of implied consent. That's why, if resuscitation is not desired, we must prove it in the moment.

How Effective Are Resuscitation Attempts?

In contrast to what we see on television, where two-thirds of resuscitation attempts succeed and a person quickly returns to full functionality, the odds in real life are quite different. Only one to three percent of resuscitation attempts in hospitals succeed; only two to six percent succeed outside hospitals. About half of resuscitated people experience significant functional impairment after resuscitation.[68] Dr. D suggests that five percent of resuscitation recipients make it to hospital discharge.

From figures such as these, it appears that resuscitation is a highly questionable bet for elders or anyone near end-of-life—a bet that could leave the recipient in worse condition than if resuscitation had not been attempted, due to damage caused by the resuscitation process itself, or damage sustained during the event leading to resuscitation.[69]

As complex as the above considerations may be, another grave, sometimes shocking aspect of DNRs revolve around the ethics of honoring or not honoring them, especially in regard to the notion of patient autonomy regarding treatment. Understanding the ethics of resuscitation is as critical as understanding that hospitals provide bodily repair, not care. With understanding comes more realistic expectations, which can serve as a buffer from extrinsic shock when surprising events occur.

The Ethical Gray Zones Around Resuscitation

WHAT ETHICAL GRAY ZONES? DNR means *do not resuscitate*, right? And the family talked about this around the dining room table a year or two ago, didn't they? It's very simple: if the patient's heart or breathing stops, the doctors cease treatment immediately. Right?

Wrong.

Having gone through the terminal hospitalizations of two parents, I have experienced three distinct DNR snafus[70] that exemplify unexpected, extrinsic shock-inducing ambiguity into situations we believed were clear-cut.

Do We or Don't We? (Extrinsic Shock/DNR Snafus #1 and #2)

What if a loved one is already hospitalized and on life support, with an untested possibility of recovery?

I have mentally labeled the circumstances around my mother's treatment plan described in this chapter's opening as DNR Snafus #1 and #2. They exemplify unexpected DNR circumstances, each with large emotional consequences caused entirely by extrinsic shock—shock that could have been prevented with adequate forecasting.

The need for patient-families to make crucial decisions ought to ensure that the decision-making process will be supported by the medical system. Support means advance notice that a decision may need to be made, a review of the range of possibilities subject to deliberation, and the opportunity to deliberate in advance of some vital choice point.

It seemed that what we really needed to specify for Mom was a *conditional* DNR. A cardiac DNR. A DNR that said "if my heart stops, do not resuscitate, but if I can't breathe, proceed with respiratory resuscitation." That's what I had presumed was in effect until I asked the fateful question. But the doctor's order didn't say that, and I'm not sure that hospital staff are ready or able to make such distinctions.

Apparently, DNR orders are meant to convey one's overall disposition regarding resuscitation. "Do me or don't do me," not "do me if this, but don't do me if that."

So the black-and-white world imagined at the dining room table, where DNR discussions relate to the proverbial "getting run over by a bus" (meaning: "I'm so injured, I'm as good as dead anyway") become very gray, indeed. How are we to make refined resuscitation distinctions before we may understand what will be involved?

The trouble is that knowing in advance, even as much as I've already described about the gray zones around resuscitation, was beyond the bounds of my family (and maybe any family). Unless one is prepared to forego resuscitation under any and all circumstances, resuscitation choices are relative, based on conditions close to the time that resuscitation could be warranted. Stipulations prior to that point can only represent generalized inclinations.

DNRs and Doctor Interpretation

Just how gray is the application of DNRs? My conversation with Dr. D added another shade: differences between doctors' interpretations. Dr. D wrote that in his view, DNRs are effective when people die, that is, their heart stops beating or they stop breathing. Implicit in this statement is that they die on their own. Dr. D further differentiated by adding that if a patient stops breathing as the direct result of a procedure he's doing, he will introduce respiratory technology whether or not the patient is a DNR. In this view, the doctor has an ethical requirement to restore the patient to his or her pre-procedure condition, because the doctor's own actions directly caused the patient's deterioration. After all, doctors are not trying to kill their patients.

Operate or Die (Extrinsic Shock/DNR Snafu #3)

We thought, after going through the DNR wringer during my mother's demise, that we were DNR pros and had encountered every problematic issue around resuscitation. It turned out that another complexity was in store for us. This one was extraordinarily profound. It arose without forecasting, and it foreclosed the last opportunity available to try to solve my father's medical problems. It represents a multi-faceted problem that I'll describe in detail.

> EXTRINSIC SHOCK AND DNR SNAFU #3: OPERATE OR DIE
>
> After two weeks of debilitation, the docs finally determined that Dad's swollen, excruciatingly painful wrist was not a new instance of cellulitis (swelling of a limb caused by water retention, a side effect of certain medications), but rather an infection.
>
> Now there were two infections: the wrist and the bladder. We believed the bladder infection came from being catheterized through the penis.[71] Such infections are frequently

caused by this procedure, and Dad had never had prior bladder problems.

Dad's wrist required draining. Great care had to be exercised due to his heart condition. In the nineteen years since his first heart attack, Dad's heart muscle had atrophied significantly. He was living on one-third of the capacity of a normal heart, kept alive by what I came to recognize as chemical life support: the morning fistful of pills.

The docs considered and dismissed the two less invasive options for anesthesia during the draining procedure (a local anesthetic and a nerve block). Dad would have to go under a general anesthetic.

We all said OK, let's do it. No question. The treatment plan was to treat the wrist infection and see if Dad's innate strength returned, allowing his system to send into remission infection two, the hospital-caused bladder infection.

Dad had one criterion: no intubation. He did not want to end up intubated for an extended time like Mom had.

A small family, we three were entirely congruent. Dad, Judy, and I were ready to sign any additional release from liability that Dad's stipulation might require. Judy and I shared Medical Power of Attorney status, and we were the sole survivors and sole heirs.

It was operate or die.

The anesthesiologists refused to operate under Dad's stipulation of no intubation.

AS EVER AND ALWAYS during each of my parents' demise, the family was provided zero forecasting. We were castaways, washed over by whatever wave of informational flotsam we found bearing down on us.

Over the phone, the lead anesthesiologist was generous with his time, and I asked him about intubation during this type of surgery. He said it's almost never required, that more *typically it occurs post-op. That yes, my father would be aware of being intubated because in order to pull the tubes out, they need first to bring a patient up into consciousness and ask a few simple questions to determine that the patient is oriented.*

That answered the question I'd been asking myself, which was, "Can I pull a fast one on Dad? Should he need post-operative intubation on the way back to consciousness, can we do it regardless of his directive?" The self-evident answer was absolutely not; there was no way I'd lie to him and risk him awakening in a condition he explicitly did not want.

Since the anesthesiologist had said he would not conduct surgery with the no-intubation stipulation, I asked if any of his colleagues would under these conditions. He asked his peers, called back, and reported that no one would do it.

I asked why not—what was the problem? He said it violated the core medical principle, "do no harm," that if they could save a life by using intubation and were prevented from doing so, they would be doing harm.

I said, "Wait a minute! He's a DNR! You mean that if he dies on the table from a cardio infarction,[72] *that's OK with you, but if he dies from respiratory failure immediately post-op and the entire family has released you from having to intubate—which is a life-support procedure—that's not OK with you?"*

"Yes, that's right," he said.

Talk about extrinsic shock! *We thought patients had some degree of control over their treatment aside from refusing or submitting to it wholesale. We were being told that refusing* part *of the proposed treatment was not a patient right.*

And that was that. Dad's future was foreclosed. There was nowhere left to go. We couldn't operate, because they refused to do so with Dad's no-intubation stipulation, a decision Dad had made (as was his right). He would succumb to infection, heart failure, or both. In that moment, I was alone with my father's death sentence.

I thanked the doc for his time and attention, and I returned to my family. It was late Thursday afternoon. Fully aware of hospital time, we needed to apply for hospice intake in order to transfer Dad before the onset of the weekend, or else he'd languish in pain and delusion for another three to four days.

Ethical Slicing and Dicing

We were in no way prepared for this.

The anesthesiologists' willingness to let Dad die by heart attack but not by respiratory failure felt like ethical "slicing and dicing," a hair-splitting distinction between acceptable non-heroics and unacceptable non-heroics. Was it? For now, let's believe that it was, as we did at the time, and as I have in the years since Dad's death, despite learning more about how surgeries are conducted.

Had the family been provided forecasting, the impasse would not have occurred at that time; it would have occurred a day or two earlier, when we all could have parsed the ramifications with less stress and the relative relief of some time to consider alternatives. It would also have been mid-week, and we could have deliberated without the pressure of another looming weekend.

At the moment of impasse, we needed one of several things:

- The anesthesiologist to query his patient-family and explore the reasons for Dad's stipulation, perhaps offering other options
- The anesthesiologist to act according to medical ethics by assisting us in finding a replacement who would do the procedure according to the patient-family wishes
- An ethics consult.

But the anesthesiologist, head of his department, offered nothing. And no one had advised us that such a thing as an ethics consult existed, let alone informed us of any resource to provide it.

This is where my earlier dismissiveness came home to roost. We had, in fact, been given this opportunity, but I had not recognized it.

A week earlier, a patient liaison gave me her card and offered her assistance. Had I taken it, we would have had an RN involved who would have helped us consider situations like these, who would act as a bridge between the medical staff and the family and sleuth out options to resolve the impasse, presumably in advance of actually needing to select one.

S INCE DAD'S DEATH I've spent a great deal of time examining aspects of the impasse and the juncture it embodied. The issues colliding at that moment present one of this book's strongest lessons.

Having lived through the ethical gray zones of DNR interpretation during Mom's intubated demise, it was ironic to go through a similar, though ultimately more painful, recast with my father. Because Dad's case was more open-ended than Mom's. If he could draw upon his innate strength and rebound from the wrist infection, perhaps he could walk out of there.

> *HIS WALKING OUT OF THERE WAS CENTRAL TO MY PLANS for his last phase of life. He had begun making noises about moving back west to Colorado. We wanted him near us in Boulder, a jewel nestled at the junction of the great plains and the Rocky Mountains. We—myself, my sister (living an hour away on the far side of metro Denver), and my wife (with whom Mort had a warm bond)—had periodically encouraged him to move out and be close enough that we could drop in on him easily, where his remaining life would be integrated with ours.*
>
> *We knew it would take some time for him to resolve Mom's passing. By the end of a fifteen-month mourning period, he had sold their condo and moved into a newly-built assisted living apartment. Despite the proximity of a fleet of cousins, in-laws, and Boomer generation relatives in Florida, he was coming to realize that no one was going to offer him the care and companionship that his two children would.*
>
> *I had envisioned running across him scootering through the neighborhood grocery store. Of meeting up at some restau-*

rant he'd discover as he scooted his way around and made our
town his town. A string of concluding man-to-man moments
under the mountain backdrop.

Fifteen months after Dad died, I telephoned the patient liaison RN whose help I had declined without even asking for it. She pulled up Dad's hospital record, and we talked. I learned that during Dad's hospitalization, the facility did not have an ethics committee, although a fledgling one had been formed since.

She opened Dad's chart, and we discussed his medical history during his end days. She said that he likely manifested a bloodstream infection and that these were common in the elderly. It appeared that the infection lodged in his wrist; bloodstream infections usually wash up into one joint or another. Due to his weak heart function, he probably would not have survived, even if he had undergone surgery to drain the infection.

We'll never know what would have happened. The tragic part is that we could have had information about likely outcomes rather than the no-exit situation we were in. A year later, clinical ethicist Diann Uustal introduced me to the term *forecasting*, giving me a name for what we lacked during Dad's (and Mom's) hospitalization. Diann also offered a name for a path we might have chosen after the anesthesiologists foreclosed the operation. It's called a *time-based trial*.

Keeping Options Open with Time-based Trials

We could have kept Dad's options open had we proceeded with the surgery with relaxed stipulations in place, stipulations that both the patient-family and doctors might have all agreed to. Here's what should have been offered. The offer should have been made by the anesthesiologist, by a doctor in charge of the treatment plan (had there been such a doctor), or by Judy or myself. Remember, at that time the patient-family was under the mistaken impression that ethical slicing and dicing was the only issue occurring. Had we understood the situation then like I do now (and will shortly reveal), the below conversation would still have taken place, but with some minor modification:

"DAD, THEY WON'T OPERATE without the intubation option, which they say is highly unlikely, seldom required, and when required, is only post-op to help you come up. If intubation is required, you'll know about it because they'll need to begin bringing you to consciousness to ensure you're OK before removing the tube. I know you don't want this, but let's make a deal. We proceed without restricting intubation...wait, let me finish...if it becomes required, let's all decide right now on a maximum duration. You tell me what that duration is. Let's find out the minimum duration the anesthesiologist will agree to. And, should you end up intubated, at the end of that duration, be it an hour or a day, I as your Medical Power of Attorney will direct that you be extubated and moved to hospice. We'll direct this in advance, so the docs know our parameters. This way we get the best of both worlds, and we get to see if you might make it out of here. What do you say?

To this day, I regret that I did not think to bring forth the time-based trial option. As an advocate, I failed in the moment.

The situation can be seen in two ways. On the one hand, my father and I had experienced a good life together: we understood each other well and had grown into a good relationship. Neither Judy nor I had any unfinished business with our father. Almost any time was the right time for this eighty-four-year-old widower with multiple infirmities to pass on; he'd expressed the desire occasionally. On the other hand, he never exercised that desire (and he could have, as we'll explore in chapter 9, "The Option to Die in PEACE"). Rather, a simple option with the potential to extend his chances, which might have placed him near us as his life closed, had been foreclosed.

The Intersection of Provider Viewpoints and Resuscitation: More Gasps Regarding Ventilation

There are yet more aspects to resuscitation and its role in treatment.

One arose early in my research. The first professional I interviewed was an acquaintance, a no-nonsense male emergency department (ED) nurse who had spent three years as a clinical manager and nursing supervisor before returning to bedside nursing. I queried Nurse N about the anesthesiologist's claim that not intubating during respiratory failure, despite the presence of a DNR and specific intubation releases signed by all the family, would equate to an abdication of the do-no-harm ethic. His assessment was that:

- The anesthesiologists' stance was based on legal-ethical grounds which carry, in the worst case, criminal and civil liabilities
- Established laws both govern and guide decisions doctors make in providing treatment; that a jury could rule against the doctor(s) were a court case to be filed
- Especially in regards to anesthesiology (which I'll summarize as essentially shutting down a human organism, then turning it back on again), monitoring and control of respiration is a central and obviously crucial part of an anesthesiologist's job
- In this context, a heart attack is clearly distinguishable from respiratory failure.

A year later, as I continued researching the intersection of DNR status and treatment, a second revealing view surfaced, this time from Dr. D. If he were extubating a DNR patient and respiratory failure occurred, he would re-intubate and convene the family for a treatment conference. He would do this because the patient, already on life support, failed due to his actions in that moment. (This example describes my mother's condition and the issues around her extubation attempt.) He would also consider the situation in light of the treatment plan. In Dad's case, the no-intubation rule was at odds with the treatment plan. When surgery is agreed on, the goal is to come through it successfully. In the medical view, that goal legitimizes the full range of medical intervention for the duration of the procedure. Our directive against intubation conflicted head-on with the treatment plan, potentially putting the surgical team in a no-win situation. According to this view, Dad's stipulation against intubation was senseless.

Like a moth to the flame, for more than two years I have periodically circled back to this DNR snafu; I've always felt that something was not adding up.

Attempting to resolve the conundrum has required repeated exchanges with Dr. D and Nurse N. While some uncertainty remains (because I cannot go back to that moment to re-interview the anesthesiologist), I have enough confidence in what I've deduced to present it here. It's important to understand, since this DNR snafu seems like a showcase example of the pitfalls that occur when we do not fully understand the intersection of a treatment plan, resuscitation matters, doctor autonomy, and patient-family directives.

For more than two years, I considered DNR snafu #3 to be ethical slicing and dicing. It made no sense. It denied patient autonomy. It seemed that the doctors using life support technology assumed the freedom to deem it part of routine treatment whenever they chose. And the doctors reserved the right to unilaterally proclaim death by heart attack acceptable but death by respiratory failure unacceptable.

Every four or five months I'd probe this issue. Perhaps I couldn't fully understand what Dr. D and Nurse N were telling me. Finally, in response to yet another query from me, they provided information different enough from our previous exchanges to cause an "aha" moment.

All along I've been under the impression that there were three possible ways to conduct the wrist drainage surgery: under a local anesthetic, a nerve block, or under general anesthesia. I've been wrong.

It turns out that there are *four* ways to anesthetize during surgery, for there are, at least, two approaches to general anesthesia—*the parameters of which were never explained to us*. Intubation appears to be the default. Intubation is, in fact, a treatment modality during surgery. General anesthesia puts a patient far enough down to require mechanized breathing assistance. Intubation is a preferred method, because the tube has a balloon at its leading end that is inflated to prevent the back flow of gastric materials into the lungs (aspiration), a very unwelcome potential problem that can lead to drowning. The fourth way, a variation on general anesthesia, is to use a Laryngeal Mask Airway, which is not often used because it does not protect against gastric backwash.

So, intubation is literally "standard operating procedure." As soon as the patient is sedated, s/he is intubated for the duration of surgery. As surgery concludes the patient is brought to, extubated and rolled out of the OR and into Recovery. If all goes well there, after some part of an hour or so, patients are returned to their hospital bed to convalesce. During the interval in the recovery room, reintubation is possible (according to Nurse N, this occurs in his ED about once per week). Further, under certain conditions, typically with the elderly, patients may remain intubated when moved from the OR into Recovery, to be subsequently extubated there. Additionally, one of the forms patients are required to sign prior to surgery will suspend any DNR directive for the duration of the surgery, to be effective upon entering the OR suite and extend until the patient leaves Recovery and returns to their hospital unit (or longer, perhaps as long as forty-eight hours post-op, depending upon the hospital).

This is all routine. And it fits with a responsible interpretation of the intersection of DNR directives and physician-induced treatments affecting respiration—assuming you agree with an all-or-nothing approach to curative treatment segments.

I surmise that when the anesthesiologist heard Dad's stipulation of no intubation, he thought, "I can't do my job without intubation, and the request is unreasonable, for it's equivalent to tying my hands at best, and asking me to assist in a patient's death at worst." I think the doctor thought that we knew that general anesthesia equated to intubation for the duration of surgery, since he told me that it was required only post-op. I now suspect he thought my query was about *re*-intubation; I don't know, and never will. I do know that this apparent miscommunication persisted throughout two separate telephone conversations, before and after he queried his colleagues.

Nobody explained to my family that surgery under general anesthesia requires intubation for the duration as a fundamental, necessary part of the procedure. We had not gotten close enough to the time of surgery to have been presented any forms to sign (including the temporary suspension of Dad's DNR, which I feel confident would have stimulated another examination of the intubation issue).

And I failed to say, "Doc, if we don't do this, all that's left to us is to roll Dad into hospice to die." I was assertive enough to engage the anesthesiologists, but in retrospect it seems—shockingly—that I failed to go the distance on my father's behalf.

A T THE TIME, WE WERE IN DISBELIEF. The docs seemed not to accept that if a patient arrests, s/he has died,[73] and that a patient choosing to not be resuscitated has a right to curative treatment up to the moment that they arrest, assuming they've stayed on the curative path rather than opt for palliative treatment or hospice. This contrasts with medical policies through which, it seems, doctors insist that we do it their way or no way at all. Aren't patients supposed to have the final word regarding what treatment they will or will not undergo?

Doctors are within their rights to refuse certain conditions; doctors cannot be forced to do something they don't want to do. Yet, establishment views and policies that change life-support technology into routine treatment, or to very tightly bind resuscitation to a particular treatment, seem to remove patient choice granted to each of us by law. *We couldn't consent to treatment about which we were not informed.*

No matter which side of the debate one is inclined towards, the anesthesiologists left us midstream. They incompletely explained the reasons for their stance, failed to offer to replace themselves, and failed to offer a time-based trial. They neither offered nor suggested any other course of action for us to take to resolve the problem. They did not ask what we might do next based on their refusal to proceed with Dad's stipulation, or what would become of us. Neither did any other provider on the case.

And what of my father's role? During this time, Dad still manifested periods of lucidity. He was totally aware in choosing hospice and abandoning the curative path (albeit misinformed about the surgery). So my regret is tempered in knowing that he knew what was happening.

I remain conflicted because I will never know for certain where he stood. Judy and I didn't ask, and he didn't tell us. Despite manifesting occasional lucidity, his capabilities were compromised. Events unfolded and we waded through them together as best we could at the time, without the benefit of what I've learned during the years that followed.

Can Do-Not-Resuscitate Directives and Orders Be Denied as a Matter of Policy?

Can DNR directives expressed in Living Wills and DNR orders expressed via state forms and bracelets be denied as a matter of policy?

It's amazing how many questions emerge from a prolonged look into resuscitation. While waiting for a friend in the lobby of a campus health center, I idly read through the patients rights placard. Three-quarters of the way down was an entry saying that DNRs would not be honored. This piqued my interest, so I called the center's medical director.

I was told that the policy was based on the age of college students. By and large (but not in all cases), any college student with a DNR would be either mentally unbalanced or too sick to be on campus (but in the latter case, they wouldn't be around the clinic, would they?).[74]

I proposed a hypothetical situation: an elderly lady, assaulted at a bus stop outside the clinic, is rescued by passersby, who bring her in. She's wearing a clearly visible state-issued, serialized DNR bracelet. After she's inside, she arrests. Would clinic staff initiate resuscitation? The director had no answer.

Other pertinent questions go unanswered, including what about white-haired professors or administrative personnel? Campus visitors? Was the policy meant to distinguish between DNR directives and DNR orders? As I write this, the center is investigating and may rethink the policy.

As to whether or not it's legal to willfully ignore DNR directives or orders by policy, I don't know. Some hospitals may refuse to honor them. And adding to the grayness around resuscitation is the hospital requirement to suspend all DNR orders during surgeries and for up to forty-eight hours after surgery.

Chalk it up as another question to consider asking if resuscitation matters loom large for you.

Future Resuscitation Choices

WHAT DOES THE FUTURE HOLD in store for those of us who may have to make resuscitation decisions?

According to a current article,[75] doctors are uncovering yet more clinical proof that death is not an event, but rather a process that occurs over time,[76] especially on the cellular level. Although an event such as sudden arrest might not be reversible, some cellular *processes* are if intervention occurs in time. Recent medical advances have shown that better managing the reintroduction of airflow to the cells of the heart and brain could result in more instances of successful resuscitation, where success is defined by return to unimpaired, full functionality.

The article discusses cases of unexpected cardiac failure and nascent procedures that retard cellular breakdown by inducing hypothermia. Quick chilling protects vital body organs from deterioration, and the subject is gradually warmed over several days while oxygen intake is carefully monitored at lower levels than are common today.

This is relevant to our discussion, because increased chances of successful resuscitation may impact how we feel about subjecting ourselves to it should the situation arise. At this writing, not many hospitals have the equipment in place to chill people (a process which must be done within a very short time frame to offer any degree of success).

Conditions and odds will change as more hospitals acquire chilling equipment. Meanwhile, what can we take away from our look at the nature of resuscitation today?

Resuscitation Conclusion and Recommendations

Do not let the issue of resuscitation go unexamined or unaddressed. Prepare the suite of Power Documents, submit them, and verify that they are in effect. Especially do not let aspects of resuscitation as applied to your specific case go unexplored. You will lose control over your patient-family destiny. By the time you regain control, you or your loved one may already have been subject to extrinsic shocks, spur-of-the-moment announcements that can rock you to a standstill. Or to massive medical interventions (resuscitation itself) and its aftermath. Or conversely, by sticking to your no-resuscitation guns, you may foreclose reasonable medical options with the potential to extend your loved one's productive life. In either case, engage all providers in this conversation early and understand the parameters of your loved one's treatment plan. Be especially wary about institutions with blanket policies ignoring or voiding patient choice regarding DNR status (ask early on to discover this). If an emergency lands your patient-family somewhere that forces full-code status on

**all, and this is against your outlook and wishes, find an insti-
tution that *will* honor your directives and move your loved one
there *immediately*, or as soon as his condition stabilizes enough
to allow transport—no matter the cost or apparent disruption.**

I suggest that any time a patient is about to leave a hospital unit
to enter hospice, three sectors ought to convene in a treatment
conference: the complete treatment group, including all attending physicians and hospital providers; the hospice intake team; and the patient-
family. Depending upon circumstances, a fourth party, an ethical advi-
sor, might be included as well.

If institutional protocols existed to provide a treatment conference
at the juncture of my family's hospital-to-hospice decision, we didn't
know about them, and they certainly weren't implemented. The hospice intake process didn't include an inquiry beneath the surface of the
family's hospice decision. No hospital representative came by to query
our decision. Not even Dad's primary care doctor (his admitting physician) offered any meaningful guidance when he finally got her on the
telephone for a final, pre-hospice consult.

Even with the DNR status decided upon and in effect, don't end up
where we did. Here are my recommendations:

- Know your values and your loved one's wishes regarding
  resuscitation.
- Put your resuscitation status documents into effect. Submit copies of the signed Power Documents, verify that they have been
  charted, and make certain that all attending doctors and nurses
  know about them.
- Do not accept a "don't ask, don't tell" hospitalizaiton. Your
  patient-family is entitled to clear, far ranging communication
  about your loved one's case, treatment, prognosis, and options—
  including, and *especially,* regarding the intersections of resuscia-
  tion and treatment matters. Actually, your patient-family *requires*
  this, and providing it is not an exceptional requirement; the core
  medical and legal principal is known as *iniformed consent.*
- If your loved one has a clear limit excluding a medical procedure

from their treatment plan (such as my father's no-intubation rule), find out in advance who among a surgical team would be impacted by that decision and interview them right away. Find out if they would be able and/or willing to comply with that stipulation. If not, ask (1) why not and (2) if they are willing and able to replace themselves. Have them give you a comprehensive explanation about the procedure and any life-support technologies routinely used during it.

- If applicable, consider negotiating a time-based trial.

- Seek, find, and utilize all the resources at your disposal before you need them. With the help and experience of people trained in medical ethics, forecast your loved one's scenario every 24–48 hours. Like a periscope, look around corners to see what is not readily visible. Expose the choices that will most likely accompany each possible outcome of whatever procedure is underway, being considered, or planned.

- Honoring patient-family advance directives and obtaining informed consent is, generally, enshrined in medical ethics and codified in law. If institutional roadblocks exist where your loved one is hospitalized, and family-focused ethical assistance doesn't exist there, move your loved one to an institution that will honor patient wishes and provide good ethical consultation (remember to identify who pays the cost of moving). Have the lead doctor on your loved one's case provide the names of other hospitals at which s/he has privileges and see if they have an available bed.

- If you think your experience in a given situation represents medical error due to mis- or non-communication, be prepared to cite industry regulatory bodies such as the National Institute of Medicine and The Joint Commission (upon which hospital accreditation and Medicare/Medicaid payment eligibility rely).[77] Citing industry regulations indicates a no-nonsense orientation that tends to prompt people to pay attention and view your grievance seriously. For situations that have become this egregious, you should already have engaged the institution's ethical support personnel.

- *Your patient-family is part of the system.* While I feel that providers and institutions have the predominant responsibility to inform their patient-family customers about resuscitation matters in their entirety, *we have a responsibility to inform providers* of our orientation toward resuscitation. Openness may beget openness. Otherwise, events will likely unfold based on unexamined and unarticulated default positions.

Remember that resuscitation status depends upon one's age and condition, patient-family viewpoints, the providers on the case, and the institution in which your loved one is bedded. Resuscitation issues are not black and white—they are very gray indeed.

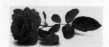

Resuscitation Recap: What You Can Do

If your loved one is hospitalized, document everything throughout each day and night. Maintain notes (your personal "chart") or keep a journal.

Be an effective question-asker! *Start now.* Has this chapter answered all your questions about:

- The relationship between treatment goals and resuscitation decisions?
- The distinctions between DNR directives and orders, and how to verify either are in effect?
- Exactly what happens with and without effective DNRs?
- The importance of learning every doctors' interpretation of his or her responsibilities at those intersections where procedures and treatment goals have an impact on resuscitation decisions?
- The ethical gray zones governing the application of DNRs?
- How doctor prerogative, treatment goals and protocols, and institutional policies regarding resuscitation may limit patient-family autonomy and choices?

If you do not have all the information you need, write your questions down. How will you get them answered? Reread this chapter? Internet research? Library research? Consulting with family and friends? A phone call to a professional or organization? Go online or pick up the phone book, find a likely contact, and send the email or place the call.

SECTION 3 | **THE IMPERATIVE TO CHANGE END OF LIFE**

W E HAVE TOGETHER EXAMINED the nature of hospitals and hospitalizations, with a particular focus on understanding and protecting ourselves against detrimental, unanticipated impacts on patient-families.

Hospitals, physicians, and the related cast of providers play a vital and respectable role in our lives. They are ever-present when we need them, and in many instances we are grateful for their accomplishments on our behalf.

This does not change their shortcomings, or our experiences due to them, nor our felt responses when enduring those experiences.

Since we are part of the system, it behooves us to ask ourselves what we want and expect of the rest of it. The medical world practically pulses with internal initiatives to change. Yet, hospitals are pounded from without by a public clamoring for reform, trying to resuscitate this nation's medical system because the system itself manifests ill health. We may want to ask ourselves how much change is possible, and whether or not incremental changes will fundamentally transform the system into something it currently is not.

Hospitals will provide a hospital experience. How can they not? Expecting something different is like going to a roadside diner with gleaming stainless steel counters, very sharp knives, and a preoccupied staff, with the expectation of eating a five-star meal. Even if the diner is redecorated with a warm motif and its staff trained in attentive customer service, in the end our overall experience of the meal will be a diner experience, not a gustatory masterwork.

Dying in an institution will yield an institutionalized death. How can it not?

We are part of the system, and we are the part that can most readily change our experience. Doing so requires that we understand fully what is at stake—because even more things happen during institutionalized dying than we've uncovered thus far.

We have to talk about death. Straight on. Is doing so distasteful? Scary? A depressing drag on happiness?

Perhaps it is at first. Just like anything we don't want to discuss...like some personal problem between spouses, friends, or adversaries. For as long as we don't discuss the problem, it sits there in the pit of our stomach or the set of our neck, shoulders, and jaw. Weighty tension intrudes on our life. Until finally we let it out and deal with whatever conflict may ensue (sometimes not any!). Then, we are relieved.

So, too, with discussing dying and death. By opening the conversation and engaging with where it leads, we can and will relax. We can, to mix metaphors, get the weight of the unspoken thing off our shoulders and instead try it on for size, considering which approach may feel right. We can loosen the set of our jaw with the fluid of our thinking and feeling. By speaking openly about death with one another, we can gain a fresh appreciation for the lives we are living.

Section 3 presents an uncompromising look at death from a physical, emotional, spiritual, and practical perspective. Here, we'll consider our options going forward.

Chapter 8, "Death Looks Like This," offers a discussion of death as I experienced it during my father's hospitalization. Every aspect of effectively managing hospitalization evolves from the possibility of losing a loved one during it. Everything presented in Section 2 is thrown into sharper focus when reflected against the one-way mirror that death may be likened to. Try as we might, we cannot view what's beyond that boundary.

The metaphorical glass does, however, reflect where those who have trod to it have been.

The trouble is in seeing as we go. The phrase "smoke and mirrors" seems apt; when living through our loved one's institutionalized end days we may not see clearly what's happening, even when our nose hits the glass. Chapter 8 tries to help you see more clearly than my patient-family did.

Chapter 9, "The Option to Die in PEACE: Patient Ethical Alternative Care Elective," introduces, examines, and offers enablement for an alternative to enduring institutionalized dying. This hugely important topic equates to moving the metaphorical mirror out of an institutional setting and into a personal one. Our place and time of death is, in fact, movable, and with very good reason: the nature of what our loved one's end days reflect back to us in our subsequent memories.

8 | Death Looks Like This

MY WIFE FLED MY FATHER'S DEATHBED—*fled his corpse*—after a scant moment in the room. She walked in, immediately exclaimed, "That's not Mort!", turned around, bolted, and was gone.

Their respective absences were utterly different. When Deborah ran from my father's body, I knew that she was still part of this world. Dad's absence was cold, absolute, and incomprehensible. He was...dead.

FOR THOSE IN ACUTE NEED OR CRISIS

WITHOUT FORECASTING, unless you've already experienced a human death, you may not recognize the behavioral and physical symptoms of its onset. Providers may not advise you of the symptoms of possibly impending death. If not, a listing of the signs is available from any hospice facility or can be found online.

By familiarizing yourself with these behaviors and symptoms, you might gain several precious days in which to COMMUNE WITH AND REQUEST TREATMENT DIRECTION FROM YOUR LOVED ONE. If you fail to do this, you run the risk of having to make a life-and-death, pull-the-plug decision yourself.

The stakes are absolute. Death is not sleep. It's the irreversible replacement of life with...what? Certainly not the life that was formerly lived beside yours.

EVERYTHING IN NOTES FROM THE WAITING ROOM EVOLVES FROM DEATH'S UNCOMPROMISING REALITY. Death cannot be undone, nor can your loved one's end days. American culture tries to deny death. We can't, of course, and time flies (even hospital time). If we don't use our loved one's lucid moments to commune together, we lose them forever. Based on personal experience, I suggest it's easier (although still very hard) to initiate unvarnished conversations about life-and-death matters with your loved one than it is to order their treatment stopped when you know that doing so is their death sentence -- or so it feels.

Depending on where death occurs, the family may subsequently interact with one or more entities, including the hospital morgue, county coroner, mortuary, alternative burial protocols, and governmental agencies. To avoid last-minute stress, once it's clear that your loved one will die, consider making these arrangements several days in advance. I know: it's awful to contemplate attending to these details while your loved one lies dying. It's your call, which will depend on the particulars of your and your loved one's circumstances.

Why an Accurate Depiction of Death Matters

Death is not sleep. Death is the unalterable inverse of life.

We accept, as part of our environment, that the people around us think, feel, move, and are conscious. Sentience and nuanced animation are part of our moment-to-moment experience. We unthinkingly accept its presence. Unless we're philosophers, we don't question human consciousness; we just interact with dozens of conscious creatures like ourselves all day long, every day, year in and year out—including our loved ones—until their sentience, and the animation it fuels...stops.

It is important to have an accurate view of death in order to protect and best utilize irreplaceable moments during the days or weeks immediately preceding the death of a loved one. An accurate depiction of death matters precisely because of the distinction between my wife's absence and my father's absence after his death. It matters because understanding that distinction informs your choices in your role as personal representative. *Knowing* that distinction, holding it close, will support your resolve to do all you can to protect the opportunity for moments to commune with and receive direction from your loved one while those moments are still possible.

You *protect* precious moments by:
- Being there to oversee your loved one's treatment
- Insisting on and obtaining regular forecasting from the treatment group so as to minimize the risk of emotional shock from surprise turns, announcements, choice points, and decisions
- Knowing the behaviors and symptoms associated with the onset of death.

You *use* precious moments by:
- Communing with your loved one
- Receiving direction from your loved one regarding treatment choices, including life-and-death choices
- Making sure your loved one's pain is effectively managed
- Making informed, ethical treatment and executive decisions on your loved one's behalf.

Knowing what death is really like is not possible unless you've experienced it up close. The best I can do is attempt to describe death using language clear enough to cut through the fake Hollywood images we are inundated with.

Even as movie and television depictions of death are paraded end-lessly, the public is shielded from pictures of actual corpses. Enter the internet, where numerous pictures of corpses are available. In my experi-ence of viewing them, even photographs do not portray death's reality as I experienced it. Photographs do not capture the irrevocable disappear-ance of your loved one's life force from this world, or from your world in particular. Although I can't explain why, photographs fail to convey how much of a *thing* a non-sentient body has become.

I had no idea what I would encounter when I entered my father's hospice room twenty minutes after his passing. I had a complete void of expectation, an absence of experience to relate to. It turns out that void and absence are two defining elements of death.

I had experienced the passing of several pets, and we've all seen dead animals outdoors. I had zero preparation for witnessing my father's body, and it shook me.

Death's finality is unlike any other ending. The finality makes the preceding days or weeks all the more important. All the problems my family experienced during both parents' hospitalizations contributed greatly to lost opportunities for communion and communication while each parent was alive.

I could offer multiple analogies for how absolute the loss of a loved one is. Each would be abstract, perhaps poetic. These would not serve our purpose here. Rather, I will try to factually describe my experience of my father, dead.

My Father's Remains

THE VISUAL IMPACT OF A DECEASED HUMAN BODY IS PROFOUND. Without feath-ers or fur, the skin predominates. Especially the face. The phrase "deathly still" applies especially to faces. If anything at all emanates from a dead face, it is the absence of the life that was formerly present.

The skin, normally rosy, takes on a colorless, gray pallor (although corpses of people of color, due to their pigmentation, may lose less color than Caucasian corpses). The facial surface literally and figuratively shrinks. A waxy tautness emerges, as if parchment were stretched over a frame. The skin goes cold to the touch with no chance of reheating. Lips once full recede. The blood no longer circulates; the heart has irrevocably stopped. There is no movement of air through any part of the body. No movement of eyes; no twitch, flutter, or blink. No movement. There—is—no—movement. This is not the apparent stillness of sleep. Sentience is gone. Spirit is absent; maybe elsewhere, maybe not.

For the first time, you may truly understand the power of life force. You know it by its complete and irreversible absence. Your loved one will not, ever again, be of this world. This person will not, ever again, grow a millisecond older (although the body's biology keeps working as its systems slowly continue shutting down). Your loved one's future has ended. Your future with this one—the person who was there a moment ago—is foreclosed. Whether the relationship was filled with love, dislike, or even hate, whatever worldly future remains is now singular—yours alone, no matter the shadows and echoes of your loved one's former presence.

The body of your loved one—for all your life an expression of purpose and responsiveness, of initiation, intelligence, and emotion—has become a carcass, a *thing*, for which there is no use. This *thing* was your living breathing loved one a moment ago. Unnerving. Unfathomable.

Your loved one's shell will never return to life on earth. At best, it will be respectfully handled. Traditionally, it will be painted, dressed and boxed, or perhaps burned to ash. Newer treatments of human remains include mixing ashes into a concrete form to be placed under the sea and become a "reef," or pressurizing some of its ashes into a precious stone. Maybe the body will be wrapped in a sheet and buried, sans coffin, in a natural field graveyard with a flat stone as a marker, or no marker at all. Perhaps the body will be plastinated[78] and displayed; perhaps freeze-dried, shattered, and used as compost; else buried, entombed, or disbursed. It might be used by science, left to decompose for forensic study, or employed as a crash test dummy.[79] Wondrously, perhaps one of its internal organs will be sewn into a live human. A human *being*. A breathing, thinking, feeling, living human being...unlike your former loved one.

THE NURSE HAD REPOSITIONED HIS BODY. His limbs were straight, the top sheet folded and smooth, tucked under his arms. I was grateful for the care implicit in her having done this.

Unless running his scooter at speed with a silly grin and a gleam in his eye, my father had moved in almost dreamlike slowness during his last years. I used to joke, in all serious-ness, that I couldn't "keep down" with him, couldn't move as slow as he did with his walker. I would have had to walk beside him as if I were doing a strange new form of tai-chi, the Chinese slow-motion meditative exercise.

How could I fathom such stillness?

I took hold of my dad's hand. It was his right hand, the one men offer each other in greeting—and parting—the hand I couldn't touch during the past several weeks, the hand attached to the infected wrist that caused him agony before being accurately diagnosed. I stood there, stunned. Trying to feel what no longer existed.

Were this a novel, or poetry, I'd say I stood "insensate." The truth is, only dead remains are insensate. We who remain here, sensate and feeling, feel the absence of the life they have relinquished.

I felt as hollow as Dad's remains were void of spirit.

I felt all the more hollow because I suspected during that time that our family's only chance for a different outcome had been wrongly foreclosed.

Years later, despite repeated pondering including a review of Dad's medical records and numerous conversations with providers, I will never know if he could have recovered and lived another year or two, possibly back in Colorado.

Spirituality and Corpses

ALTHOUGH I AM NEITHER ORIENTED TOWARD NOR SCHOOLED IN spiritual prac-tice, I recognize that certain readers may be. I cannot disallow the pos-sibility that the deceased's spirit may hover near the body or continue to inhabit it for some days (nor can I disallow the possibility that nothing exists after death beyond memories carried by the living).

How we experience and describe death reveals much about our worldview. Mine tends toward the pragmatic with an element of the spiritual. For me, this has evolved as an appreciation of the equanimity and sagacity embodied by some who engage in spiritual practice, plus a willingness to accept supernatural experiences as valid. I did not discern latent elements of spirit or of the sacred in the body, as some who follow spiritual paths describe, although my worldview and orientation did not predispose me to believe in or sense spirit in the deceased. Should spirit reside in the deceased, it is orders of magnitude quieter than what they manifested in life. Even if my experience included manifestations of the spirit lingering, that would not change the fundamental absence of a formerly sentient loved one. Thus, I focus on the temporal, the worldly. And the clinical nature of hospitalized dying is nothing if not worldly; hospitals are not spiritual environments and are not conducive to spiritual nourishment.

The worldly experience of hospitalization and hospitalized dying certainly contains emotional and spiritual lessons. For families experiencing death for the first time (or second), I believe the lessons are understood retrospectively, as the result of soul searching and mentally reliving the experiences.

Whatever spiritual gains may ultimately be had by the departed, or perhaps even we who remain, we still must endure the physical reality of a loved one's death.

What Might You Encounter?

THE CONDITION IN WHICH YOU ENCOUNTER A LOVED ONE'S REMAINS may differ according to various factors. The primary factor is where the patient was at the time of death. According to an emergency department doctor, if someone dies in the ED, catheters and IVs will likely remain for some time, until a coroner sees the body. If a person dies in their hospital bed while under curative care, if the catheters and IVs have not previously been removed, they may remain for some period of time, or may be removed by the attending nurse. If in a palliative care environment (hospice or home), the mechanical hookups will be absent and whatever clothing was worn will remain.

According to Dr. L, if the patient has died during a resuscitation procedure, the body will be stripped completely. Dentures, if present, will be removed. Nurses will try to clean the body, perhaps including a sponge bath, then (usually, but not always) cover up the exposed body with a sheet before family arrives.

Not long after death, the body will feel eerily cold, even before it cools to room temperature (a body at room temperature feels absolutely icy to the touch, since our brain expects a body to feel warm).

Traumatic deaths are different, and an ED doctor may advise the family not to view the body of a loved one who has died of an accident or homicide.

The important thing is that this is *your* loved one's remains, and viewing them is your decision. You can view and be present with the remains or not, whichever best supports your own closure. You can ask a nurse or doctor what you will see and to cover the remains to any degree you prefer. In any case, if in the hospital, expect to be ushered along sooner rather than later. They'll want to move the body to its next stage and free up the bed.

The Psyche Must be Fed

IN AMERICAN CULTURE, WE TRY TO HIDE DEATH—and to hide *from* death. Yet regardless of how we might try to deny death, it remains a part of our psychological makeup, of our psyche. Denying psychological reality is like trying to starve a part of ourselves that needs nourishment. The psyche will rebel. It must be served; it must be fed. If real nourishment through real experience is withheld, psychological junk food served up through fake experience will have to do.

If the number of deaths discussed and depicted in our media and films is any indication, our communal psyche has a voracious appetite. According to my comparison between my father's remains and the depictions I've seen, with one exception, all the depictions look fake.[80]

I don't have personal experience with how dead faces change over time. The body goes through a well-known progression as its systems begin shutting down, death occurs, the body continues shutting down, and decay begins. From my research, which includes perusing many pictures of the dead, their faces seem to look more lifelike hours or days after death than my father did twenty minutes after his. Perhaps it's because pictures are inanimate to begin with. Perhaps it's impossible to capture the loss of sentience except through direct experience.

It could be that the state of my father's remains was transitory. Having never seen a human die, I can't address the moments immediately prior to death, the moment of passing, or the minutes that immediately follow, during which the face must change. Occasionally movies try to depict these moments, usually in a fanciful or horror setting.

My sister, however, was present at my mother's passing fifteen months prior and arrived at Dad's bedside shortly after I did. She said Mom looked the same as Dad, with the same characteristics (albeit more pained, indicating the nature of her particular end-of-life ordeal).

The deluge of Hollywood death depictions feeding our national psyche begs for an examination. For now, let's merely acknowledge it as a rain of false images that substitute for real experience.

Caregivers I've spoken with suggest that people whose illness results in a slow final decline may literally look more dead than alive in their final days, and that their appearance after they depart does not differ from their appearance as they lie dying.

One moment we have sentience—awareness and a capacity for experience. Then, suddenly, life is gone, and stillness remains. Seeing death so starkly, it is clear that we have no future with this loved one. No last chance to say or express anything.

I know the conversation I wish my father and I had had—and didn't. It would have gone like this:

The Conversation Dad and I Didn't Have

THE ROUNDING DOCTOR LEAVES THE ROOM after an examination of and conversation with Mort, during which Mort is extremely lucid, complete with the occasional repartee. The moment the doc's feet are out the door, Mort's next comment to Judy and I is completely nonsensical.

"Dad, I need you to stay with me for a minute or two. Can you come back and do that? Let's have a family care team conference."

"Yeah, Bart. Care team conference..."

"You know, without the surgery—and you allowing intubation—we're at the end of the line. You won't live, and hospice is the only alternative."

"I'm gonna get right up and dance the jig," he jokes wryly, looking at me with facetiously raised eyebrows and his trademark clownish, self-described 'shit-eating' grin. He vaguely moves his good hand in an attempt to make circles with his finger. Even this close to dying, Dad was as alive as ever.

"Oh yeah, right!"

"Bart, I wanna go home."

"You can't, Dad; they won't let you back in assisted living."[81]

Dad sighs, a resigned expression on his sentient face.

"Dad, I'm your Medical Power of Attorney, and I need you to clarify your wishes."

"I wanna be up there with your momma," he says, inclining his head upward.

"And you will. But, you know, your heart meds are keeping you going. And two things can happen in hospice: one, you decline; two, you turn around. That's a long shot, but miracles do happen."

"Miracles."

"Dad, keeping you on your heart meds seems like cross-purposes to hospice, like it will prolong your death..."

"Stop the meds," he orders, interrupting me.

"...but we can hope for a miracle and keep you on them for a day or two. If there's no miracle, we can stop the meds then. Or, you can opt out, quit the heart meds now, and guaranteed, you'll see Mom sooner rather than later. What do you want for yourself?"

"I wanna call it quits, Bart. I'm done."

"Does that mean you're ordering your hearts meds stopped now?"

"Yeah."

"Dad, this is a life-and-death decision, and I want to be really sure. You want to stop the heart meds and opt outa the miracle?"

"Yeah, we'll call it a day."

...

"Dad—jeez, love you, man!"

"I love you too, Bart."

"Dad, thank you for everything you've given me throughout my life. I'm gonna miss you. I was looking forward to you living near us. I wanted that. I regret that we won't have that opportunity. I know you'll wake up a few times in hospice, so we'll be there to see you when you do, OK?"

"Yeah. Give your girls the big squeeze for me."

What follows is a crazy attempt to hug each other, with me leaning over, trying to avoid his infected wrist, Dad trying to return the hug using his one good arm entangled in IV drip lines and other hookups.

"Yeah, and give Mom an amorphous squeeze for me, too. A real infusion, eh?"

Dad smiles in appreciation of my offbeat associations, a characteristic of mine that he implicitly understands. That he understands without explanation exemplifies what we lose when a loved one dies: one of very few fellow humans who know us so...intrinsically.

The Conversation Mom and I Didn't Have

Fifteen months earlier, my mother and I didn't have a conversation either. Unlike the above wished-for scenario, the conversation I didn't have with my mother was because intubation made it impossible for her to speak.

IT HAD BEEN ABOUT TWO WEEKS that Ruth lay intubated, unconscious in the ICU. Occasionally she'd move slightly or moan softly, but there was never any rise to consciousness.

Due to the length of time she had the breathing tube inserted into her trachea through her throat, a decision was looming to either authorize a tracheotomy or acknowledge her demise and "let" her die.

Despite family hand and voice contact with her, she made no response and initiated nothing…

…until one day when I was the only other person in the room. Suddenly, she came to and voiced something—or more accurately, tried to voice something as best she could with the vent down her throat. She had a pained look in her eyes and on her face.

I thought then, and I believe now, that her activity was completely and directly conscious. I didn't know then, and I don't know now, what she was trying to communicate.

I moved right up by her and responded with something, probably on the order of, "Mom, I can't understand you." My intention was to begin posing questions to try to ascertain what she knew and verify what she wanted to say.

But her availability was momentary. As quickly as she had come up, she slipped down again.

I don't know what disturbed me more: her distress, my inability to understand, or that neither my father nor sister (two people whose love for her were not burdened with unresolved emotional complexities) were with her instead of me. In any case, that irreconcilable moment was the last interaction I had with my mother.

Signals that Death May Be Near

WOULD YOU RECOGNIZE THE BEHAVIORS AND SYMPTOMS associated with impending death? Would you recognize them in enough time to come to grips with the possibility and to use whatever diminishing opportunities presented themselves to commune with and seek treatment direction from your loved one?

My mother was for practical purposes comatose, on life support from the moment she entered the hospital. We were not caught off guard by her death. However, Judy and I didn't recognize certain of Dad's symptoms as hallmarks of impending death. We thought debilitation, not the onset of death, was their cause.

I can no more undo my failures than I can bring my father back for a second run-through with the benefit of what I've learned in the years since his death. This weighs on me, like carrying a stone.

Metaphorically, I pick this stone up, wave it around some, lay it down again, and begin the cycle anew. This mental activity mirrors one of the physical manifestations of dying that was not forecast for my family during Dad's end days. It's called "picking the air," and it is apparently related to behaviors such as picking at bedding or clothing.

PERIODICALLY THROUGH THE WEEK, Dad had been moving his arms around above his torso. Occasionally he'd include commentary. "Bart, help me move these. This needs to go here, and these things go there."

At the time I had no idea what was happening. There were no things to move. I didn't know that the dying "pick the air," or that psychologically oriented, perhaps spiritually attuned, healthcare providers interpret this activity as one of several the dying engage in, in an apparent effort to resolve whatever aspects of their existence the activity might represent.

One day, I realized that Dad would keep doing this until whatever he was trying to accomplish was accomplished. We shared the trait of being efficient packers. We could each maximize the efficiency of space, be it for storage or to support varied activities.

Intuitively, I decided to help him. I couldn't know for certain what lay behind Dad's actions. Rather than play a game of pretending to move imaginary items, I simply said, "Dad, you're done. It's all moved."

"I'm done?"

"Yeah man, it's all put away. You got it."

"I did it."

"Yeah, you did."

"Good."

And that was that. The end of my father's picking. Not mine, however. Every now and then I mentally pick at my memories, grasping for resolution. My thoughts and spirit get heavy like stones, dense with the remembrance of absent forecasting and what I might have done had I known earlier what my father's symptoms meant.

Back then, by the time I figured out to search the internet for "dying symptoms" and found hospice websites listing them, at least three if not five days of opportunity with my father had slipped past. During that time his condition worsened, his availability diminished, and my sister's and my distress and confusion deepened.

My regret is not the errant remorse of absent relationship. It's not the result of a belated attempt to resolve at a deathbed the unresolved interpersonal junk that keeps people apart from one another—stuff that often entangles families and the treatment group alike as a loved one lies dying, further burdening an already multi-layered event. My remorse revolves around my failure, as Dad's Medical Power of Attorney and son, to know enough to have helped him to the best degree that I and medical technology could have. My remorse is about the simple communications that did not transpire between our patient-family and the treatment group throughout Dad's demise.

Now, at the very least, I can help you avoid pitfalls and the losses associated with them by summarizing the main symptoms of impending death.

The Symptoms of Impending Death

In my experience, the symptoms of impending death typically present over a period of weeks. How to ascertain whether a particular symptom actually portends the possibility of death or is associated with deep stress is beyond my limited experience.

Each death is unique, and there is no specific timetable. In some illnesses, people decline in a linear way; in other illnesses, people can decline and rebound cyclically.

There is disagreement about the meaning of certain behavioral symptoms of impending death. Those who believe that sentience and spirit die with the body may accept common clinical interpretations (for example, that confusion means dementia). Those who believe that life transcends the physical plane and continues in a nonphysical realm after the body dies may make a very different meaning (for example, what looks to us as confusion is the dying person completing unresolved life issues or seeing beyond the earthly plane).

Although a deep examination of these distinctions is beyond the scope of this book, the meaning you make of your loved one's behavior is central to this discussion. Do your research, mull it over, and come to your own conclusions. Your loved one will approach their death their own way, no matter your viewpoint. But with your own forecasting of these matters, you'll get to decide whether or how to engage them on their final journey.

The lists below are not comprehensive. You can find more information including the widest possible range of symptoms by perusing a variety of hospice websites and literature. Also, be sure to ask your loved one's treatment providers to help you interpret behaviors that arise in your specific case. The point of the list, in the context of this book, is to forecast what dying typically includes, so that if and when your loved one exhibits any of these symptoms, you won't be taken totally by surprise, misinterpret them, and lose valuable opportunities for communication and communion.

Behavioral Symptoms of Impending Death

Behaviors come and go. Nurses may not encounter particular behaviors associated with death due to not rounding frequently enough to be in the room when the behavior manifests. When you, your loved one's personal representative, are at the bedside, you may want to ask the nurses when to expect people to round. If you experience these behaviors, don't make the mistake we did and just assume their cause is debilitation. Alert the providers so they can assess your loved one's state should they manifest:

- Delusions (misconceptions of reality which are contradicted by what others perceive)
- Hallucinations (hearing, seeing, or feeling things not present)
- Picking the air (repetitively moving the hands or arms around)
- Speaking in symbolic language, for example, about "packing bags" when referring to preparation for death
- Diminished self-restraint, exemplified by the story below.

MORT HAD BEEN BEDRIDDEN *for about ten days when suddenly, one afternoon, he decided to exercise...a rational move, since he'd been lying around for a long time.*

He decided to exercise nude.

This wasn't hard to accomplish; his wardrobe consisted of a hospital gown. He couldn't get it off, so he just shoved it up. There he lay, complete with a urinary catheter and IV drips, and proceeded to lift and lower his legs, all the while accompanying his movements with verbal descriptions of them.

Aside from this instance, my father did not lay around doing exercises. The spectacle was unusual, yet perfectly understandable. Unless the body is seriously shutting down, it needs to move. Nudity was either the only option (as the gown constrained movement) or simply the absence of everyday self-restraint.

And, when was the last time you spent ten days immobile, or even several days without once getting naked?

I was inclined to let him be. My sister's sensibilities differed from mine. Failing to persuade Dad to cover up, she sought assistance from a unit nurse, who also failed, Dad rejecting her interference (he kicked her out.) At this point, I gave voice to my own assessment that what Dad wanted was normal, but the context was abnormal. The environment allowed only very limited choices. We left Dad alone to do his own thing. We were not there to usurp his authority, but rather to extend it.

Physical Symptoms of Impending Death

Unlike transitory behavioral symptoms, physical symptoms associated with death may be more evident. Most of these become prominent during the very end days, known as active dying:

- Less physical activity and movement
- Diminished interest in one's surroundings
- Diminishing interest in (actually, need for) food and water
- Lowered body temperature
- Lowered blood pressure
- Diminished circulation to the extremities, which begin to cool and turn splotchy from the blood pooling
- Diminished speaking and verbal responsiveness
- Dry mouth
- Shortness of breath
- Grayish quality to the skin color
- Fingernail beds become bluish
- Coma
- Reddish-brown urine
- Breathing changes: a pattern of several rapid breaths followed by a period of no respiration at all (referred to as "agonal respiration")
- A rasping sound to the breathing known as the "death rattle" (caused by fluid in the airway)
- Cessation of breathing

Handling the Body

AMONG THE THINGS THAT OUGHT TO BE FORECAST in a hospital during a potentially terminal hospitalization is the need to make arrangements for what to do with your loved one's body after death occurs. If this is not forecast, expect to be advised directly after death that you'll need to make arrangements to have the body picked up and removed within a short time frame—so short as to infringe on your grieving. This pronouncement serves as one more instance of institutional disregard for the family's overall experience.

The protocols after at-home deaths (often referred to as "unattended deaths") may vary from state to state. If your loved one dies at home, the authority you'll need to deal with is the county coroner's office in the county where death occurs.[82] The coroner may want to view the body and determine the cause and manner of death. The coroner will "certify" the death, and only then begin processing the death certificate. In some locations, a hospice nurse will come and certify the death.

If your loved one dies in the hospital, the doctors will certify death. Unless circumstances fit certain legal requirements, you won't have to deal with the county coroner. Traditionally, however, you do need to select a mortuary and provide its phone number and contact information to hospital personnel so the mortuary can be called to come collect the body.[83] If you haven't selected a mortuary, the body may be taken downstairs to the hospital morgue and kept there until a mortuary is chosen and their pick-up vehicle arrives.

A mortuary is the intermediary that is legally required to arrange the body's disposition, be it cremation or burial. The need to select a mortuary is yet another aspect of end of life in hospitals that is not forecasted. If your loved one's impending death is certain, take the initiative and add this task to your to-do list and begin making arrangements prior to the actual death. Hospitals don't like to keep the dead around very long, and you'll likely feel pressured if you wait until after death to attend to these tasks.

The mortuary will provide you with original death certificates (you'll want plenty of them for settling the estate[84]) as well as your loved one's remains in whatever form you desire them.

One Hospital Morgue

During my mother's demise, a family lost their daughter to complications from childbirth. The family's cultural group was one in which mourning included keening. This public, mournful wailing was, of course, a breach of hospital decorum, and security staff was called to quiet them.

Afterwards I ran across a security guard in the hall. We recognized each other, since I'd been cruising the hospital for well over a week. She was the same ethnicity as the family of the deceased, and it had been personally difficult for her to quiet the keening. She wanted to support the family but had to enforce hospital rules.

She asked after my mother and inquired as to whether or not we had arrangements in case she died. She then looked around, lowered her voice, and told me confidentially to be sure to make prior arrangements to have her body removed rather than allow the body to be taken downstairs to the hospital morgue. Remains, she said, were not treated respectfully down there.

It was ironic that the only forecasting we received during two terminal hospitalizations occurred by chance through a security guard.

Funeral Arrangements

IF YOUR FAMILY HAS PLANNED for or desires a conventional funeral and burial, mortuaries ("funeral homes") are the businesses to contact. If your desires are unconventional and do not include cremation, the county coroner's office is one place to learn what is allowable in your community.[85]

In general, there are two basic scenarios: what's known in the trade as pre-need contracts or advance resting arrangements, and the making of arrangements near or at the time of death. Given how mobile our society is, whether or not to preplan burial may depend upon such things as where a spouse or adult children live, the existence of a family plot, etc.

A pre-need contract typically includes basic body disposition and a memorial service. It's all arranged for in advance, so in the event of the death of the named person, you call the mortuary and they provide the services specified in the contract. The difference is that you don't have to search for and decide upon a mortuary. If a pre-need contract is made with a national mortuary chain, the family will have access to mortuary facilities nationwide. This means that if an elderly loved one dies in a sunbelt retirement state, but a service is desired in the state where various survivors live, this can occur at no additional cost (aside from transporting the remains).

Veterans and the disabled children of veterans are eligible for interment at any Veterans Administration (VA) cemetery that has room.

My father had made prepaid local cremation and memorial arrangements and had planned for burial at a new, nearby VA cemetery that was under construction at his time of death. Mom's ashes were in his closet. We had no desire to bury them two thousand miles from our home, so Judy and I had their ashes shipped across the country. They were interred at a nearby VA cemetery, in the earth, in a short plot the VA uses for cremains.

Upon settling the family estate, I came across a pair of pre-need contracts from a mortuary chain that my dad evidently had forgotten about. These contracts are transferable. I called the mortuary, presented the necessary papers, and transferred the contracts into my and my wife's names.

Changing Our Experience of Death

CAN WE ACCEPT DEATH? On the face of it, this is a silly question. We certainly can't prevent death, although we try to stall it through heroic medical intervention.

It takes involvement as a personal representative in only one person's demise to begin understanding death (which is quite distinct from viewing countless fake depictions of death).

Ultimately we will accept death because we must. The question becomes, can we accept death so as to make our experience of a loved one's end days less painful than they become when we try to deny death?

This we can do. Without therapists. We begin by talking openly and candidly as friends, families, and as a society. Once we start this conversation, options other than an unthinking pursuit of hospitalized dying may open up for many of us.

Expanding the range of options for where and under what conditions we die is imperative. Doing so requires that we examine some things we take for granted or don't even know occur.

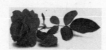

Death Looks Like This Recap: What You Can Do

If your loved one is hospitalized, document everything throughout each day and night. Maintain notes (your personal "chart") or keep a journal.

Be an effective question-asker! *Start now*. Has this chapter answered all your questions about:

- Why it is important to have a clear and accurate view of death?
- What death really looks like?
- What are the typical behaviors and symptoms that precede and accompany death?
- What becomes of the body after death?

If you do not have all the information you need, write your questions down. How will you get them answered? Reread this chapter? Internet research? Library research? Consulting with family and friends? A phone call to a professional or organization? Go online or pick up the phone book, find a likely contact, and send the email or place the call.

9 | The Option to Die in PEACE: Patient Ethical Alternative Care Elective

D EATH IS TRULY SENSELESS. *I do better when I can make sense and meaning of events. Last Tuesday, upon hearing of Mom's terminal diagnosis, I spent some time at Eldorado Canyon State Park. This is a transitional place, where the Rocky Mountains relinquish themselves. Sheer rock walls tower 1,200 feet above South Boulder Creek and the plateau stretches beyond into an infinity called the Great Plains.*

This cold, solitary day felt like a metaphor for what Mom's condition had been the entire week prior: hopeful elements advancing and retreating over a chill backdrop. In the canyon, moments when the icy breeze stilled felt less bitter; moments of sunshine and warmth offered transitory hope for the day to fundamentally change. I stood there, focusing on the apex of this place, scanning the cliff face and its heights, until I became aware of the creek beside which I had trudged, and then I noticed its nature.

It was amazing. It was a unity and a diversity—all water, but in many different forms. Ice slabs inexplicably lined the creek side, as if placed there in preparation for laying some bizarre ice patio. The creek was partly frozen and partly not;

water flowed below the ice in some places and above the ice in others. Slush lined the shore. Rich shades of translucence, transparency, and opacity appeared, changing as sunlight reflections changed with each step or shift of focus. The creek-canyon air was moist, a relief from Colorado's inescapable dryness. Somehow, I could feel a hint of warmth...a fitting, though elusive, metaphor for where to seek a gateway to healing upon the loss of a loved one—especially upon the first instance of death in my immediate family.

This place spoke to me in a manner reminiscent of Rainer Maria Rilke's The Sonnets to Orpheus. *I was standing in a reflection of the inscrutable relationship between time and life and death, which Rilke so beautifully portrays in every sonnet. Here, time was time, flowing water was a human lifespan, frozen water was Rilke's impenetrable "unsayable sum"[86] of moments, and the slush in which I stood was the indeterminate place we inhabit in our desolation.*

I thought, "I can accept this. I understand that Mom is not so much leaving as she is going, that her eighty years here was tangential...a full lifespan by our experience, yet but a brief cosmic moment. A moment we've shared between the stuff from which she came and the place where she has gone to what moments remain—an "unsayable sum" of moments.

~ Comments Excerpted from My Mother's Memorial Service

FOR THOSE IN ACUTE NEED OR CRISIS

THE MOST EFFECTIVE WAY TO MANAGE a terminal hospitalization is not to have one, or to escape one as quickly as possible.

This is not a glib assessment. Adding to our examination of the kinds of experiences any hospitalization can include, this chapter offers surprising information from several medical disciplines and A FRAMEWORK FOR CHOOSING TO OPT OUT OF TERMINAL HOSPITALIZATION.

Revelations from medical anthropology, insight from a physician-ethicist, an interesting statistic from hospice, and this author's reframe of what constitutes heroic action combine to create a "container" supporting the choice to die a non-hospitalized death.

I call that choice The Option to Die in PEACE: Patient Ethical Alternative Care Elective.

THESE ARE AMONG THE MOST SENSITIVE OF SUBTOPICS under the shadow of death, itself a topic virtually taboo in American society. A notes-page summary cannot begin to offer enough for you to fully contemplate making a personal choice to die outside what has become the

default national norm. Thus, if opting out of hospitalization may apply to your loved one and your circumstances, even those in acute need or crisis should take the
time to retreat and read this chapter in its entirety.

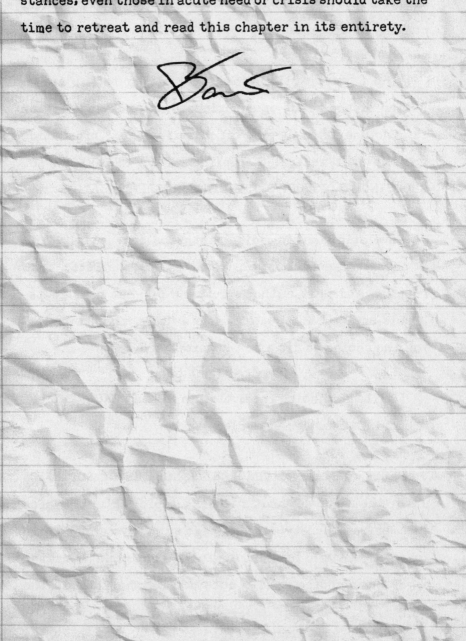

ETERNITY HAS BEEN DEFINED as a progression of endless *nows*. In other words, eternity is nothing more than an endless succession of moments.

What fascinates most about our experience of moments is how elastic each can be. Some moments seem tauntingly fleet and others achingly long. Perhaps a long moment is actually many moments in which nothing changes. As we've seen, in the context of *Notes from the Waiting Room*, long moments in hospital environs can accrue into lost opportunity, unless you're aware of their potential meaning.

The interface between life and death, wherever it occurs, makes for the most poignant moments. It's clear to me, both in the abstract and from my experiences, that end of life is a time when our humanity ought to govern; that technology, public policy, and institutions ought to serve humanity rather than humanity serving them. Or worse, serving as fodder for them.

Our humanity deserves the best we can do to support it. Each of our lives is ours alone. Our humanity resides in our experiences. How each of us experiences our own end of life matters more than how some hospital or treatment protocol plays out.

The fact that more medical options exist than ever before in history provides for the possibility of incredibly joyful moments. When overdone, those same medical interventions can needlessly create poignant moments that exacerbate tensions and remorse.

We all know that it's overdone, that the "machine" tends to take over. The term *machine*, with its demonic undertone, really means "system." Early in *Notes from the Waiting Room*, I commented on "the system." I listed ways in which the system manifests during end times, including our beliefs, values, and ethics; family dynamics; cultural milieu; and medical, legal, and political entities. You and I—*we*—are part of the system. *We* share responsibility for our outcomes.

Systems are not static, and the healthcare system is changing. This book is one attempt to encourage change among the treatment-seeking public, through a deep understanding of what occurs, and by making explicit what is implicit during terminal hospitalizations.

New initiatives are being introduced in various sectors of the healthcare world as hospitals and providers attempt to solve some of the systemic problems we've discussed. A growing movement to formalize palliative care within hospitals is one indicator of the system changing; in 2006 the American Medical Association recognized palliative medicine as a subspecialty.[87] This, and other reform efforts, concentrate on improving the experience of hospitalization. Maybe it will all get solved during my lifetime, perhaps thirty-five years or so. Maybe not.

These efforts are vital, insofar as they go. Or rather, from where they start: during hospitalization. While we ought not minimize them, we must recognize that efforts by the system to reform itself do nothing to change the fact that dying in a hospital will yield a hospital experience, subject to the values of a high-tech, command/control, medical system that seems to be wholly uncomfortable with death. If we don't want to die in a hospital, we must advocate for something different.

Whatever advocacy I advanced on my parents' behalf pales beside the advocacy that we must champion to reform end-of-life experience for the majority of our citizens. We need to do this so that each of us can exercise an option to receive humane medical assistance without having to enter the hospital. In this chapter I introduce a new option that has many benefits for individuals and our society as a whole. I call it The Option to Die in PEACE: Patient Ethical Alternative Care Elective.

Examining end-of-life options challenges every part of the system, including *ourselves*. Near this book's beginning, I wrote about a metaphorical pond, by which I meant an environment in which participants get immersed and even onlookers become saturated. I used this metaphor to describe the intellectual challenges that understanding terminal hospitalization represents. I stated that *anybody standing on the shore of the metaphorical pond is bound to get wet. Anyone navigating its waters will get spiritually tossed.*

Further along I introduced the metaphor of the crucible and its heat, by which I meant our *experience* of the hospitalization, our felt response to all the overlapping agendas within the compressed time frame of a terminal illness and demise.[88]

Allowing, devising, and supporting humane end-of-life options represents yet another voyage across the metaphorical pond to yet another crucible awaiting us. The waters of this voyage and the focus of this crucible are inside our hearts. On this personal voyage, distinct from the public voyage a hospitalized demise represents, both the waves and the temperature are lower. And the horizon stretches farther.

What follows presumes that the essential nature of hospitalized dying will not change, despite insiders' reform movements. My assessment is that, in general, they are too cautious, too slow, too bound up in their own institutionalism. I propose an alternative. In order to understand it, we need to understand the system as it exists today and reach some conclusions—some of which may be startling.

MY IMMERSION IN THE METAPHORICAL POND began several weeks before my visit to Eldorado Canyon, when I learned of my mother's collapse. I had read and resonated with Rilke's sonnets a decade earlier. *The Sonnets...* succeed in bringing some of death's mystery into life. Never did I expect to *live* that poetic mystery, as I did in Eldorado Canyon. The world suddenly embodied the unknowable essence of Rilke's masterwork. That remarkable experience helped me accept my mother's imminent passing. It helped alter my perceptions regarding life and death. I'm very clear that this occurred because I wanted it to occur; upon my first reading of *The Sonnets...*, I longed to experience the unfathomable nature they present, to know both sides of the divide—to see beyond the mirror.

Consciously sensing something of the beyond is a privilege. Doing so without *starting* the experience in an altered state is notable. I experienced a glimpse of the nature of death and its relationship to life while alive.

I was not the one dying. But, of course, we each will encounter death. How do we change our assessment of death's relationship to life, and our approach to dying, in enough time to ensure (insofar as is possible) the peaceful death many, if not most of us, desire?

Based on my experiences of hospitalized dying and my suspicion that the medical system cannot overcome its inherent problems and humanize death inside hospitals, I want something different for myself, my extended family, and especially for my nuclear family. Arriving at that place is the focus of the remainder of this chapter.

Existing End-of-Life Options

LET'S REVIEW THE OPTIONS for dying that currently exist for us.

Sudden Natural or Accidental Death

Those who die of a catastrophic health failure or an accident are gone in a moment. Obviously we have little or no control over this. Whether peaceful or gruesome, those who die immediately, and their survivors, need not worry about the matters we are discussing.

Suicide

Those who are desperate or unwaveringly resolved may take their own lives. With luck, they will not endure agony beyond that which drives them to suicide.

Euthanasia, Assisted Dying, or Self-directed Dying

Few societies provide help in ending one's life. The Netherlands and Oregon are two places where provisions exist for help in certain cases. Eligibility is strictly governed, and guidelines exist for the types of help that are legal. Oregon requires that a six-month (or less) terminal diagnosis be given by two physicians. Reviews are built into the eligibility process. An individual requesting physician-assisted dying must make multiple requests separated by a minimum of fifteen days. Eventually, medicine that will end life within a minimum of three hours is prescribed and delivered to the individual, who must consume it him- or herself.

We'll discuss below the notion of self-directed dying and how it reframes this sensitively considered manner of death.

Deaths that Occur in a Planned Manner

Some diseases lend themselves to known timelines, given certain deviations that are also generally known. Cancer is a prime example. It's not unusual to be given a terminal cancer diagnosis six months or more prior to death, while still in good enough condition to remain active. Some cancer patients enter into a hospice plan that provides morphine patches worn on the skin. With this pain management, the patient can continue to enjoy physical and social activities until his or her condition further deteriorates.

Dying in a planned manner makes dying outside the hospital feasible. With such a long dying trajectory, one can plan well in advance and, assuming access to the required resources, select the environment in which death will occur, be that at home or a hospice facility. With this option, there should be few shocking surprises (although some shock is intrinsic to dying and death). Everyone involved will have ample time to come to terms with the dying person's end of life; the basic choice has been made, and the patient-family is no longer subject to making myriad short-range decisions as if they were a ball cascading through a pinball machine.

Dying Unexpectedly Due to a "Wrong Turn"

Wrong turns are distinguished by entrapment in a situation we would prefer had not happened. *Notes from the Waiting Room* focuses on entrapment in hospitals. This is for good reason: fifty percent of us currently die there, with the ratio poised to rise as the Boomer generation ages.

To be clear, hospitals are not jails. Any "sentencing" to such facilities is a natural result of being in such poor condition that you can't go elsewhere, or that wherever else you do go is perceived as worse than the hospital environment (e.g., nursing homes). Preclusion from returning home is especially relevant if you live in a controlled community that disallows intentional dying, or if you do not have the resources for family assistance or nursing care at a private residence.

My mother might have died of respiratory failure on the spot had she not been intubated. She didn't suffer an instantaneous fatal collapse, but apparently the interval between severe respiratory distress and placement on life support was short. Within some minutes she wound up on life support and was transferred to a hospital ICU, with no notice to her family. That occurred three weeks before her actual death, during which time we all languished in an indeterminate state.

My father's dying trajectory was grievous in its own way, quite different from Mom's. He suffered consciously for some weeks. His wrong turn was unanticipated, although not beyond expectation, given his overall condition. He chose hospitalization for routine procedures. He either miscalculated the risks or was not thoroughly advised regarding them. In any case, he unexpectedly failed coincident with those procedures. Although he could have ultimately left the hospital, his choices were reduced to hospital, nursing home, or hospice, since dying at his assisted living residence was disallowed at that time. In both events, the family existed in a state of confusion and shock for weeks, not knowing what would happen until death foreclosed all other options. All of us lived with death to some degree during those last weeks of my parents' lives.

Palliative Care

Two programs exist to provide comfort care and adequate pain relief to the terminally ill. The less formalized program is called palliative care.

To *palliate* means to alleviate discomfort without removing its underlying cause—that is, without trying to cure disease. Palliative care may be provided in the hospital, sometimes in conjunction with curative treatment. Nascent palliative programs champion care provided by multi-disciplinary teams comprised of a palliative care doctor, a registered nurse, a chaplain, and a social worker. Sometimes limited or modified curative treatments are offered under palliative care solely for the palliative benefit they may offer. The best approach to palliative care comes from doctors who carry its wholistic torch. These doctors see a return to a viewpoint of palliation as the umbrella under which all medical care is offered.

Palliative care is humane and firmly within the spirit of the Hippocratic oath. According to some mission directors, ethicists, and physicians, providing it has captured the attention of hospitals nationwide. At this writing, most hospitals do not yet offer developed palliative programs. This is beginning to change—and will require buy-in, and cooperation, by all practicing independent physician-scientists in order to change prevailing patient-family experience. In any case, if you want palliative care be prepared to specifically ask for it.

A central goal of palliation is to mitigate pain. Some curative treatments can help accomplish this, as can treatments as yet outside the allopathic mainstream (which many Americans know work through direct experience). In the context of terminal illness, pain mitigation essentially means drugs. Serious pain-relieving drugs are strong enough to dull cognition, and they are addictive. Various delivery methods are available; meds can be delivered via mouth, patch, or IV drip (with the latter under control of the patient, who can self-administer microdoses as needed).

During end of life, providers and their patient-families must balance effective pain relief against loss of cognition and against addiction. The former tends to distress patient-families who might lose remaining opportunities for communion. The latter tends to distress providers who, for reasons I don't understand, seem unwilling to be party to an imminently terminal individual becoming addicted...especially since studies show that when lower doses of opioids are dispensed around the clock, pain can be managed with reduced tendency toward addiction.

A movement is afoot to formalize pain as the fifth vital sign. Pain would join pulse, respiration, blood pressure, and body temperature as an indicator that warrants intervention to bring it into an acceptable range. Certain states (among them California) and federal agencies (the Veterans Administration) have already incorporated pain into their formal codes as the fifth vital sign.

Notwithstanding this movement, pain management is both highly individualistic and not widely enough practiced. Anecdotes describing inadequate pain relief for hospitalized relatives have appeared in various media and watchdog communiqués for years. I know of two terminal hospice patients—a friend of the family and my own father—whose POAs needed to intervene to order that their loved ones received adequate pain control even during their very final days in hospice.

Palliative options do not offset the fact that hospital deaths occur within the normal framework of hospitals that I have described. You might want the option of having palliative care *outside* a hospital setting.

Hospice

The second program providing comfort care during the dying process is established and known by some but not all Americans. In any case, it is widely misunderstood: hospice.

Hospice is a program, not necessarily a place. It's administered as a free Medicare benefit to every American who qualifies for Medicare; those who don't must be insured for hospice[89] or may take advantage of free hospice care supported by community donations. The Medicare Hospice benefit includes a range of treatments so long as the hospice program orders them. As with hospitalization, if a patient needs more frequent attention than a hospice-at-home program can provide, the patient-family will need to use its own resources to provide it. There is no age requirement for hospice care.

Hospice focuses on palliative care—and it is care in the true sense, distinctly different from curative *treatment*.

Hospice care can be received at home, at a dedicated hospice facility, or in a hospice wing of a hospital. Hospice itself is not a death sentence, and death is not hastened under hospice care.

Unfortunately, gaining entry to hospice requires that one formally abandon all curative therapies. This exemplifies the either/or framework that controls medicine. It's unfortunate, because some treatments that are primarily curative also have palliative benefit. Practically, the occasional curative treatment may be allowable (for example, the removal of a tumor that's pressing on the esophagus), and savvy doctors can sometimes code treatments that otherwise would not pass muster. On the whole, however, the hospice philosophy is predicated on the patient-family having accepted death as a natural outcome.

Admittance to hospice requires a terminal diagnosis by one physician, with death expected within six months as per the doctor's best prognostication. With a long-term disease like cancer, that diagnosis can more readily be made many months prior to death. Those with other ailments whose trajectories are not as clear-cut as cancer may not qualify for a terminal diagnosis until after they've entered the hospital and failed there. Patient-families with loved ones who fail during a hospitalization have zero time to plan for their loved one's end-of-life circumstances. Rural areas served by a hospice program located in a small city serving as a hub for the community may function with relaxed standards; a rural ED doctor told me that the hospice he consults to accepts all who come.

Although death is usually predictable by the time one enters hospice, there are exceptions to every rule. Some people with long-term diagnoses recover, leave hospice, and live for years. Some exit hospice for days, weeks, or months, and reenter when their condition deteriorates further. If a curative treatment is desired, patients can leave hospice for a week or two, pay for the treatment directly or through their health insurance, then reenter hospice care (it's OK to leave and return to hospice, repeatedly if need be). Sometimes those who are assessed as certain to die undergo a miraculous recovery and return to active living. Hospice accommodates all these circumstances without prejudice.

The following areas represent the core focus of hospice:

- Effective pain and symptom management
- Emotional and spiritual support for the patient and the family
- End-of-life closure; completing life well.

Hospice can be seen as the luxury model of terminal care, due to its humane focus on both the dying and their loved ones.[90] The entire patient-family is assisted. The shift in orientation from curative hospitalization is subtle and profound: from doing *to* to doing *for*.

Granted, physicians do not mean to dehumanize and objectify their patients. These things happen as a natural outgrowth of component management, the insurance imperative, and denying death when death cannot be denied. Patient-families themselves can be complicit in the latter.

Hospice as a Station of Last Resort

I stated above that hospice is not a death sentence. Abandoning curative treatment acknowledges impending death (be it six months or six hours away), so it's easy to understand the confusion. Adding to the confusion about hospice's role is that one-third of Americans using hospice do so as a station of last resort rather than as it is intended: a provider of humane treatment during the entirety of one's demise.

The director of one of the nation's oldest hospices showed me statistics indicating that nationally, one-third of hospice patients are customers (my word) for only seven days or less. Of those, roughly half are in hospice for only four days or less before dying.

These are revealing statistics. It means that one-third of those who learn about and accept hospice use it only for end-stage[91] assistance. They have attempted to deny death, experiencing an institutional demise of however many weeks. They've acquiesced to hospice only at the end of that experience—*when they are actively dying*—for it typically takes several days to die after curative efforts have run their course and people acknowledge that a life is about to end.

The reasons for this are both personal and institutional. Personal, in that patient-families often fight heroically until as near to the bitter end as possible and allowable. Institutional, because dying is not diagnosable or billable, only curative activity is. Thus, unless death occurs "unexpectedly" in a hospital, once cure is formally abandoned, the patient-family must find somewhere else to die.

Hospice is a flexible program. It does not turn people away. If we want to use it as a location to lie down and die, it's there for us. However, hospice is primarily available for much longer-term assistance, beginning with a doctor's terminal diagnosis months before death is anticipated. Generally, seven (or fewer) days is simply not enough time for hospice workers to help a family come to terms with the end of a loved one's life.

Hospices Are Not Created Equal

Lastly, and regretfully, all hospice programs are not created equal. In general, the smaller the chaplain-to-patient ratio, the better the care will be. Urban hospice workers can be extraordinarily overworked, making their everyday lives not too much different from their curative counterparts, hospital nurses. In metropolitan areas, larger hospices may provide better service due to their economics (Medicare pays hospice a small set fee per patient per day; patients who use fewer hospice resources subsidize those who require more; this is known as "cost shifting"). Even the largest hospices rely upon donations. From my limited discussion with hospice personnel, knowing how to select a hospice (that is, knowing what to ask) represents another education in itself. Best practice is to start your investigations well before you think you or a loved one might need hospice.

Such are the conditions under which people die. So why is another option needed? To answer this question, we need to explore what really occurs during a hospitalized demise.

The Surprising Nature of Hospital Death

NEITHER OF MY PARENTS' DEATHS WERE NATURAL. They occurred in controlled environments under controlled conditions. They died under the influence of hospitalization. By this I do not mean that their deaths were caused by hospitals, but rather that the manner of their deaths was tightly controlled by the hospital environment, both its constraints and its unspoken sequences.

How do hospitals structure our end-of-life experience? Various assumptions and values shape these critical and poignant times. Although assumptions and values underlay almost everything people do, the coming together of a very naive culture (patient-families) with an experienced, well-developed, and rule-bound culture (hospitalized medicine) during end-of-life hospitalizations may be likened to a wave slamming into a seawall, where the water must ultimately channel down a drain. Explaining these forces is the realm of medical anthropology.

An enlightening source on this subject is a book by Sharon Kaufman, *...And a Time to Die: How American Hospitals Shape the End of Life*. Kaufman, a medical anthropologist, spent two years embedded in hospitals, rounding with treatment groups, observing the demise and deaths of many patients. Kaufman articulates several core points:

- Death in the hospital has evolved into a realm all its own, a "gray zone of indetermination." At this threshold, it is possible to hover in an in-between state, neither fully alive and certainly not dead.
- Individuals and society are ambivalent about death. On the one hand, we want the "good" death, a natural, peaceful exit. On the other, we don't want our loved one to die, and we therefore approve various amounts of intervention.
- We approve these interventions, in part, because our culture values self-determination, and we expect the right to exercise that control. Yet patient-families don't possess adequate knowledge to know what is really happening, let alone to make life-and-death decisions.

Kaufman advances several illuminating points, two of which are particularly relevant to this conversation.

Death Has Been Brought Into Life

Kaufman articulates the idea that hovering in the zone of indetermination has brought death into life. This phrase describes the time period in which a patient would die without biomedical intervention, popularly referred to as "life support" by laypersons and as "treatment" (as best as I can figure) by providers. The zone of indistinction is characterized by ambiguity: continued treatment does not restore the patient to health but does forestall death.

Occasionally a case like this reaches national attention, as did that of Terri Schiavo, the clinically brain-dead Florida woman maintained for fifteen years by a feeding tube. My mother was maintained for three weeks by artificial respiration. The experience of living through three weeks of indetermination in a hospital setting introduces all the problems we've discussed so far.

The clinical notion of bringing death into life differs from bringing a *discussion* of death into our normal conversations. We must bring death into life in the conversational sense, if we are to reform end-of-life options so that those patient-families who do not want the risk of existing in the indeterminate zone are not by circumstance compelled to.

In that zone, we have a situation in which patient families—agitated, confused, and untested (dare I call them the dying initiates)—are paired with providers, members of the medical order who have seen death unfold many times. The arena is charged emotionally, morally, technologically, spiritually, and with financial and legal undertones. It is an experiential cauldron—the crucible about which I have written. Within this environment, in which *all* participants overtly fail to acknowledge death, medical personnel become subtly suggestive. They may withhold information that they know about the patient's condition, the dying process, and death because we expect (and even demand) that they prolong our loved ones' lives. They may reveal just enough to gently guide us towards making life-and-death "decisions." Such decisions are often illusory because practitioners, familiar with the onset of death, know how we must choose, based on the well-known timetable on which death generally unfolds during end-of-life hospitalizations.

Hospital Deaths are Managed and *Actively Timed*

Thus, one aspect of modern end-of-life hospitalization: the manner in which hospital deaths are actively managed. Insurance imperatives and discomfort broaching to patient-families what's obvious to providers results in a process subject to managing. This aspect of hospitalized dying is not disclosed by hospitals and treatment group members (although it's evident to anyone who has lived through it and subsequently reflects on the experience).

Another startling and highly meaningful revelation from Kaufman's research is how death is not only managed but actually *timed*. This occurs when both the family and treatment group share the conviction that either nothing more can be done to extend life or that the patient would not want to continue in whatever condition they are in. Achieving unanimity on these issues can be an understandably complex progression unfolding over days or weeks. The trajectory, however, is well known to treatment group members who have been involved in tens, hundreds, or more deaths. It's new only to patient-families who encounter it for a first or even second time (it's not like most of us get a lot of practice).

Stop and absorb the notion of death being institutionally timed. The ramifications are profound, and we'll address them in the next section.

In some, or perhaps most, circumstances, treatment providers foresee death long before they share that assessment with the patient-family. They wait for the patient-family to come to that conclusion over some days or weeks.

Reasons for this delay vary. They include valid treatment goals, patient-family expectations or desires, ethical quandaries, and providers' understandable fear of being accused of abandonment (of hastily or prematurely abandoning a dying patient-family)—a very serious allegation.

It is especially in this latter regard, the notion of abandonment, that we can help providers. By the time you've finished contemplating this chapter, you may be better prepared to meet providers as co-gatekeepers at death's door. If providers were freed of the fear of being accused of abandonment, perhaps they'd be more open to broaching their sober, and sobering, assessments of our medical outlooks during our end days.[92]

No matter the complexities (and they are many), underlying the deliberations is an undisclosed imperative to "move things along," in Kaufman's words. What this means is that patients must exhibit progress or regress but cannot be maintained indefinitely in an unchanging state in the hospital—insurance won't pay for it. There are no extended deathwatches in twenty-first century hospitals as there were as late as the 1960s. There is either treatment and partial recovery (enough to move the patient elsewhere for more complete recovery), or there is the abandonment of curative treatment and relinquishing the patient to subsequent demise (which will require that the patient be moved out of the hospital). Or, of course, a patient might suddenly "crash" and die on his own while everyone else is trying to figure out what to do or what not to do.

The imperative to move things along, subtle as it may be,[93] combined with technological interventions ultimately results in death being timed to within several days.

It's important to restate that this is the fate awaiting up to fifty percent of Americans—those who die in hospitals—a statistic poised to grow. The fact that many hospital deaths are not natural, but rather timed, is especially relevant to The Option to Die in PEACE.

Taking Control of Our Deaths:
The Option to Die in PEACE

If we do not die accidentally and do not want to die in a hospital, where then should we die? When? And how?

Just because we utilize and benefit from medical technology to extend our lives, it does not follow that the government, institutions, and doctors ought to control our dying and deaths.

I believe we share an almost universal desire to die in peace, and for our survivors' experience of our dying to be as unburdened as possible. We want the option to make death our own personal matter, not a legal, administrative, or (overly) medical matter. To the extent we want institutional help, we want that help to serve, not subjugate, our humanity.

We want pain management, without having to get a terminal diagnosis by failing utterly in a last hospitalization that we can no longer escape. We want advance eligibility for a formalized program, which we will initiate when we choose after becoming eligible. We want a new class of treatment group members to be trained to function within it. We want to save ourselves and society the difference between the modest cost of such care and the cost of that needless last, desperate hospitalization ($85,000 in my dad's case, $145,000 in my mother's, plus the unknown but doubtless significant cost of all the attending physician-specialists).

The Option to Die in PEACE

We want PEACE: a **Patient Ethical Alternative Care Elective**.

Patient here means two things: first, that people at end of life are in fact patients, working in concert with an assistive team; second, that we approach the end of life patiently, neither in a hurry to fix the unfixable nor to delay the inevitable. *Ethical* means that the option is morally palatable. *Alternative* means that we don't have to enter the hospital to be eligible for care; that humane, high-quality, effective palliative care will be provided outside of the hospital environment. *Care* means access to palliative measures sufficient to truly mitigate pain and support patient-family autonomy, delivered in a manner experienced as caring. *Elective* means that the choice to initiate care remains with individuals, not medical, legal, or political institutions, and that participation is optional. The extent of institutional involvement would be in crafting policy enacted into statutes that enable the PEACE alternative and removing any impediments that may currently exist.[94] After individuals become eligible for inclusion in the program, it is entirely up to each of us when to initiate that care.

PEACE is an option, not a mandate. Those wanting to pursue all that hospitalization has to offer, its potential for benefit and burden, would remain free to do so.[95]

Eligibility to Die in PEACE

Eligibility to die in PEACE would depend upon each individual's condition, alone or as measured, first, by seriously declining health and, second, by age. Since the goal of PEACE is to avoid a terminal hospitalization, if possible, eligibility would be less stringent than hospice eligibility currently is (hospice requires an "imminent terminal" diagnosis of six months or less by two medical doctors).

One's overall health condition alone, or in combination with advanced age, would trigger periodic eligibility reviews, much like routine physical exams or disease screenings. A person's likelihood of slipping into a terminal decline would be the unit of measure. When that likelihood edged up to a certain percentage in the viewpoint of a licensed and qualified physician, the individual would become eligible for PEACE.

Once eligible, each individual could enroll and call for assistance. At this point, PEACE becomes indistinguishable from hospice or palliative programs supervised by hospice (depending upon how close to active dying each individual is when enrolling).

The option to die in PEACE is not simply about dying peacefully. PEACE puts individuals in control of their own demise by widening the one pathway leading away from extended hospitalization, while bringing institutions and technology together in a role that supports individual patient-families as sentient beings during a most poignant time.

Overcoming the Obstacles to PEACE

WHAT PREVENTS US FROM TAKING CONTROL OF OUR DEMISE? The answers lie in personal fears and beliefs, medical bias, politics, finance, and ethics, discussed below.

Identifying and Overcoming Fears

I believe that we fear four basic things when contemplating end of life: losing dignity and control over our condition and treatment, pain, dying, and death itself.

Fear of Losing Dignity and Control

The fear of losing our dignity and losing control over our fate ought to be enough to keep many of us out of hospitals. But we roll the dice because we are programmed to live.

Having the degree of choice we do is unique and new in human history. The elders of the World War II generation are the first people to have access to a smorgasbord of life-extending medical interventions. For the half of us who die in hospitals, one or another hospitalization—

we don't know which—will be our last. The ultimate loss of dignity and control comes when we fail so utterly during a hospitalization that we cannot get out.

Loss of dignity and control includes that which is experienced by the patient (having tubes inserted or taken out, being poked and prodded, draped in only a hospital gown) and by family members (lack of forecasting, discontinuity of care, extrinsic shock, and the potential for the loss of diminishing opportunities to commune with and receive direction from a loved one).

Ironically, providers also lose control to the extent they foresee death but wait for the patient-family to come to that conclusion also.

Yet we go to the hospital because we do not yet have a widely understood, viable option to die in peace elsewhere.[96]

Fear of Pain

Today it is possible to eliminate pain in its entirety (or close to it), whether in the hospital or at home. Resistance to doing so exists in hospitals. Reasons include patient reluctance to admit that they're in pain, provider misinterpretation of how much pain patients may be in, and provider fear of inducing addiction (even in imminently terminal patients).

Fear of pain is justified. Pain can overwhelm us. It can rob us of the ability to be present with the rest of what our remaining time offers.

Fear of Dying

How much of the fear of dying is attributable to fearing the loss of dignity and control, and to the fear of pain? How much of the fear of dying would be eradicated if we could set these other fears aside? By guaranteeing the option of a pain-free demise under personal (rather than institutional) control, fear of dying would resolve to a series of existential questions; concerns of the mind and heart when contemplating death.

Fear of Death

We don't know if there's an "other side" beyond earthly sentience (or before it, for that matter). The fear of death is also the fear of the unknown. For some, it may be the belief that there is another side and it won't be pretty for them; for others, that only nothingness awaits, that they will be snuffed out of existence in a way that stuns the mind.

One option would be to believe that whatever happens after death, all will be good and as it should be, for all involved.

PEACE CAN MITIGATE THE FIRST TWO FEARS. With dignity and control maintained and pain controlled, we may have enough internal resources available to resolve the second two fears, assuming we have not already done so well in advance. The deathbed is a little late in the game to resolve these issues, unless you need the momentum provided in the crucible of impending death (although, by many accounts and common sense, even a stroke-of-midnight resolution gets the job done).

With an option to mitigate pain and maintain dignity throughout our dying process, more of our resources are available to make peace with our mortality, as individuals, families, and society. Doing so may also help us make peace with the idea of a more natural death.

What Kind of Death is Natural?

When people do not die of a diagnosed condition or accident, they are said to die a natural death or "death of natural causes."

A valid question is whether the presence of any intervention at all represents something *unnatural*. This harkens back to Philosophy 101 and whether or not the works of humanity are part of, or separate from, the natural world.

I define natural death as one that is allowed to occur without so much medical intervention that the patient dies of complications caused by the intervention (examples of complications include pneumonia, bladder infection, MRSA infection, multisystem failure after weeks of nonstop heroic biomedical intervention).

A natural death does not need to be entirely free of interventions. Natural death (inside or outside of hospitals) does not preclude the humane use of medicine or technology to relieve pain and suffering.

It is possible to die a natural death in our current world. Many Americans do. How many die comfortably? I don't know. What we do know is that hospitals are not places where natural deaths typically occur;

twenty-first century hospitals are not supportive of natural dying.

Patient-directed Dying

Patient-directed dying is a distinction championed in a book of the same name by Tom Preston, M.D.[97] Preston suggests that the common notion of physician-assisted suicide does not apply to the terminally ill—that suicide is impossible for the terminally ill, who by definition are already dying and cannot be cured. Traditionally, suicide occurs when the subject is not dying, and is either healthy or in a reversible condition. The terminally ill who choose patient-directed dying do not initiate their dying; *they complete it.* They do so on their terms and timetable, not the medical system's. If a lethal dose of medicine is provided, then those who prescribe and fill the prescription enable patient-directed dying, but they do not assist (assuming the patient takes the medicine without assistance).

Do these distinctions matter? I think so. I think they're logical within a framework of ethical considerations. Are they ethical slicing and dicing? If so, is it any different than the sort we encountered during my father's conflict with the system, what I refer to as my family's DNR snafu #3?— that a DNR death due to heart attack on the operating table is acceptable but a DNR death due to respiratory arrest post-op is not, just because the latter can be "overcome" by quickly shoving in a tube? Either death was acceptable to my patient-family under our particular circumstances. Our conundrum *was* ethical slicing and dicing, because even had we proceeded with an understandably intubated general surgery, Dad would not have wanted *reintubation* post-op, had he arrested. The medical system's values overrode ours. Essentially, the institutional argument resolves to the fact that a technology exists to keep the lungs processing air indefinitely (or until the trachea collapses), whereas an equally *convenient* technology does not exist to keep the heart pumping blood.

As medical technology progresses, we will need to parse ever finer ethical considerations—ever more minutely examining and analyzing the choices in front of us. The current technological paradigm will make increasing demands of our ability to be insightful. To what level are we willing to go? The cellular? The microscopic? How do we identify our beliefs? When is enough enough? When do we finish fighting "the good fight" for life? In the crucible, is it a good fight—or is it something else?

7 Ten-Thousandths

We bring to, and focus so much into the crucible, those last two to four weeks of hospitalization. Yes, it is a life at stake: my parents', your spouse's, any loved one's unique life.

As precious as each life is, can we gain any perspective as to the proportionality of effort brought to fighting the time of demise?

Let's make some assumptions: an eighty to eighty-five year lifespan and a three-week terminal hospitalization. Simple math reveals that the crucible represents approximately *7 ten-thousandths* of our loved one's lifespan (that's the last $7/100^{th}$ of one percent of the lifespan).[98]

To account for all our personal variables, the math is easy to do for your own circumstances: divide the number of weeks comprising a demise into the total number of weeks of a lifespan.

I bring this up not to quantify lives, but rather to throw into relief the enormous energy, angst, and tribulation experienced and dollar cost expended during these times which are brief in terms of lifespan yet long and draining in the experience of families and personal representatives.

Identifying Your Beliefs: a Zillion Questions

Earlier I said that your job as a personal representative was to ask, ask, ask questions on your loved one's behalf. When contemplating end of life, we also need to answer some. We need to pose, pose, pose questions of ourselves.

Here goes:

What kind of death do you believe to be best? What makes for a "good death"? Where do you draw the line between extending life and prolonging death? Who gets to invoke, or ignore, the ethical/religious principles of double effect and proportionality[99] that purport to balance intended and unintended, primary and secondary, welcome and unwelcome effects—the individual, one or more providers, or an institution?

Are your beliefs the same when you contemplate your own death as when you contemplate a loved one's demise? A stranger's? How are your beliefs shaped by the nature or quality of your relationships? Adherence to religious or spiritual paths or doctrines? Are your beliefs open to examination and change?

Do you believe that institutions and strangers have the right and authority to determine your time of death or your loved one's time of death? Do you believe that you should be free to?

Who should have control over life's ending? We can't turn back the technological clock. Assuming carte blanche access to modern medical treatment and a societal blank check to pay for it (a dubious assumption, as we'll see shortly), we *will* use the marvels of modern medicine to extend our lives. The question bears repeating: does it necessarily follow that, because we use modern medicine to extend our lives, modern medicine and the institutions in which it is practiced ought to have control over our deaths?

If your beliefs limit your own choices, should others in our society be similarly limited according to these beliefs, or ought they have freedom of choice over their own dying?

These are challenging questions. It's time, as individuals, families, and a society, to answer them. No patient-family's death should be subject to the mounting extrinsic shocks that the system in its current state imposes on us.

I agree with Preston that reframing assisted-suicide to patient-directed dying can inform a decision to forego or quickly cut short that last, terminal hospitalization. Death by stopping treatment is not suicide, nor is it euthanasia. It is the natural result of letting go. Making a choice to stop treatment each individual's right by law and by broadly accepted moral code.

The question is, *When does one let go?*

The surgeon, Pauline Chen, suggests an answer in *Final Exam: A Surgeon's Reflections on Mortality*. Chen describes the distinction between *living with* a disease to *dying from* the disease. Recognizing this distinction leads directly to the question, "When do the burdens of fighting this disease outweigh the benefits of not dying quite yet?"

Actually, the question is more likely to be phrased in terms of multiple diseases, because for the first time in history, we have successfully fought off enough of them, sometimes over several decades, and live long enough to succumb to multiple medical problems simultaneously.

One Peaceful Demise: An Example We Did Not Manifest

MY FATHER'S GOALS AND DESIRES WERE SUFFICIENT to cause him to break his vow of "no more hospitals" and hospitalize himself for what turned out to be the final, inescapable time.

Had our family dynamics been different, we might have come to a different conclusion and he to a different ending. Had Dad considered his adult children as full partners after Mom's death, had we adult children exhibited a bit more initiative, we might have had some conversations about his options before he entered the hospital.

We did not have those conversations. But I have imagined how Dad might have arranged things so as to die without beginning or enduring a terminal hospitalization.

In Dad's case, his heart meds were keeping him alive. He was on what I consider chemical life support (the daily fistful of heart meds). Given this state, Dad had an interesting option: the possibility of controlling (partnering with?) the nature and timing of his own death. He could have concluded that the risks of another hospitalization and cardiac interventions were too great. Since he was weakening, he could have consulted with his cardiologist and obtained a terminal designation (assuming a six-month-or-less prognosis) and qualified for hospice.

Dad could have kept on with no further medical intervention beyond eating pills, weakening as his cardiovascular system atrophied. Or, he could have stopped eating the heart pills that were keeping him alive. He would have taken himself off life support. He could, thus, have consciously timed his own death to ensure that he would never risk rehospitalization. Enrollment in hospice would have made Dad eligible for pain relief and comfort care.

Or, he could have called his primary doctor and requested the diagnosis on the basis of openly opting to stop his heart meds, a choice certain to lead to imminent death.[100]

In this proposed scenario, we would have said our good-byes. Yes, I wanted him to end his days nearby, but only if he could have enjoyed some months here. He lived a long, fruitful life. His partner of sixty years was gone. We had good, clean family relations. We could have helped him leave this world. Not without sadness, but certainly without all angst we endured during his hospitalization.

Instead of exercising these options, he rolled the dice by going into the hospital—and lost.

Overcoming Medical Bias

In *Last Rights, Rescuing The End of Life From the Medical System*, Stephen Kiernan presents a sobering view of the almost complete lack of attention to the needs of the dying.

To a certain extent, medical bias against dying—discomfort acknowledging it, avoidance of caring for dying people humanely, lack of training regarding death—mirrors society's discomfort with death. One would hope, however, that those whose profession is to minister to medical needs would move beyond this societal reluctance and manifest a more compassionate response to death, of which they see so much and therefore intimately know as every person's last chapter.

Overcoming medical bias, like other bias, begins with the acknowledgement that it exists and has negative consequences. The consequences of this denial of death in medicine are not trivial; they cut into a patient-family psyche as sharply as a scalpel into flesh. Withholding information from the patient-family that ought to be forecast (perhaps because it portends a negative outcome, even when death is not imminent) is one manifestation of this denial. In essence, withholding negative outcome possibilities that could have been forecast is playing God with peoples' psyches.

Medical curricula ought to include teaching true care of the dying, and continued medical licensure ought to require proficiency in the care of the dying for physicians and others whose specialties or practice places them alongside the dying on a regular basis.

Transferring Control

If doctors cannot learn to accommodate death as a routine part of our lives, and of their own lives as clinicians, they ought to cede control over death to those who are comfortable with it. If physicians persist in interpreting death as personal and professional failure, if they refuse to proactively engage their patient-families in straight talk, if they balk at forecasting in enough time to alleviate extrinsic shock at the bedside, then they should own up to their orientation. We need not judge them harshly for clarifying their outlook and the focus of their work. Rather, the reverse is true: denial of their outlook and focus results in harsh experiences for their patient-families and then in harsh assessments by survivors.

Others stand ready and waiting to assist the dying. Some allopathic physicians are leaving curative medicine and focusing on palliative end-of-life care.[101] Nurses and ethicists hired by hospitals to engage in ethical support within the hospital environment are ready and willing to assume formal roles in helping the United States' citizenry die humanely.

The Dollar Cost of Hospitalized Dying

It doesn't take a math wizard to figure out that families and society can benefit by avoiding millions of terminal hospitalizations costing $100,000 or more apiece, plus doctor costs. The disproportionate cost of futile end-of-life hospitalizations as a percentage of our national healthcare expenditures has been studied and is well known. It's a subject of debate among policy makers and medical ethicists. Individuals and families' life savings are at risk should they be uninsured, or if their insurance fails to cover the full costs of a protracted demise.

Dying at Home, in Home-Like Communities, or Hospice

THE PATIENT ETHICAL ALTERNATIVE CARE ELECTIVE implies home as the place of choice to die.

Dying at home is not free of angst or cost. It will not be for everybody. Some illnesses, due to their timing or trajectories, may not lend themselves to home care. A human support network is required in most cases. While no one should be forced to die at home, it's conceivable that some who would like that option might be challenged; for instance, if they do not have a family, or if family members are not or cannot be available to them during their demise. With or without outside support, caregiver stress syndrome is a real and present danger—spouses can and do die of it, predeceasing the partner for whom they've been caring.[102]

Dying at home might be impossible for the elderly living in facilities with rules prohibiting such a pathway, enforced by daily checks if the staff hasn't seen or heard from the resident on a given morning.

Perhaps we need more communal options for the elderly who are closing into life's final passage. At Naropa University's summer 2007 Integrating Spirit and Caregiving Conference, I lunched with a Coloradoan who was involved in just such an effort, helping to design a small community where dying at home is to be supported by common cause, if not covenant. These types of communities are in our future; some movement toward them is nascent.

Hospice facilities are available to the terminally ill and their families (not all hospices have facilities). Of those that do, they will vary from home-like to institutional (including wings in existing hospitals).

Reframing Heroic Action

PERHAPS THE GREATEST IMPEDIMENT TO PEACE lies in the notion of heroic action. *Heroics* describes the efforts made to prolong life during the weeks of an essentially futile hospitalized demise. Life-and-death choice points abound, and the questions defining them also define the extent of our angst. How many weeks will we forestall death? How many interventions do we try before we accept something as incurable? Do we resuscitate? If so, under what conditions? Do we ignore our loved one's resuscitation directives? What constitutes "plugging our loved one in"? Having done so, when do we—when can we bear to—"pull the plug"? Will we be killing them if we unplug them? Are they committing suicide by unplugging themselves? Whose responsibility is all this? Or, is this conundrum some unquestioned construct?

The best way to manage a terminal hospitalization is to avoid having one.

Don't go.

And if you end up hospitalized, cut it short and get out.

How do we manage *that*?

Redefining Heroics and What Constitutes Heroic Action

Heroicism[103] lies at the root of the efforts we engage in to extend life. Without much questioning, we consider heroic activity to include resuscitation efforts, plus all those activities during those last weeks of life in which we pull out all the medical stops in the hospital. This "heroicism" invokes all the forces that make this time and this experience a crucible: all the emotional, spiritual, religious, medical-technical, moral, legal, and financial factors commingling in a compressed time frame.

As we've seen, the patient-family is caught up in a bewildering scene, subject to the array of problems unique to this time and place. We've explored those problems' severe consequences.

Why engage in heroics? The obvious answer is because we don't want to die or our loved one to die. But why not, if we, if they, have lived full lives?

Less obvious answers relate to the role we give to heroicism in our lives. We may believe that it's our duty to fight to live. Some subscribe to religious beliefs regarding the sanctity of life, which governs the choices deemed acceptable.

Common to these beliefs is the largely unexamined notion that the only time and place constituting heroic action are the very last weeks of life under end-stage conditions. That's when we will engage in heroic activity to satisfy the requirements we believe we must satisfy.

But what if we have already satisfied those requirements? *What if we've already acted heroically and have done so for years, perhaps decades?*

I PROPOSE THAT THE WEEKS OF A TERMINAL HOSPITALIZATION are not necessarily the time for heroics. These weeks are beyond any requirement for heroism. They represent a final phase of life, the transition to death (if we let it be), otherwise a time of last-ditch craziness if we pursue medical technology in a hospital setting. Medical professionals use the concept of *futility*. Futile it may be; crazy-making it most certainly will become.

The very good news is that accepting a reframe of what constitutes heroics does not deny heroics, *for we have already engaged in heroicism!* We've engaged in heroic action from the moment we first fight back against our first serious ailment!

Heroics begin when we undergo our first cardiac bypass. Or hip replacement. Or dialysis treatment. Or chemotherapy. We do not give up or give in.

No matter how ordinary any of these representative procedures (and others of similar extent) may be for professionals who conduct them, they are not ordinary for individuals undergoing them. Nor are the efforts and accommodations that follow. My father's last nineteen years represent a time of increasing heroicism: a repeat bypass ten years after an earlier bypass surgery; maintenance angiograms and angioplasties; years of pill-taking, including popping the occasional nitro for cardiac abnormalities; twice-daily management of water retention by the drug-induced shedding of copious amounts of urine—a process requiring two five-hour, home-bound sessions seven days a week to stay in proximity to the bathroom (meaning that one's out-of-house activities need to be scheduled around those sessions, every day, year after year).

These and similar actions are heroic actions, and undertaking them satisfies the human imperative to fight for life and to sanctify the life we are given by Creation by not giving up on it.

During these years, everyone is heroic: the patient, the spouse who assists and accommodates lifestyle changes, the doctors who perform the procedures, the scientists who create them, the chemists who develop powerful medicines, and even the pharmaceutical companies that fund and make them available.

During these years, everybody is a good guy; everybody wears the white hat, so to speak. These are productive years, during which human bonds are cemented in memory as children become middle aged and next generations emerge into young adulthood—all witnessed, perhaps assisted, by elders whose socially productive lives have been gratefully extended by applied medical technology.

Once we stop and think about it, it's easy to see the heroism in all who persevere in these actions, year in and year out.

And one day, each person so engaged will fail. "Crash," in medical parlance. She or he will take an insurmountable turn for the worse... from living with the disease(s) to dying from the disease(s).

That day either lands our loved one in the hospital or occurs during yet another hospitalization our loved one has embarked upon. That day, we get to choose what to do, and what not to do. That day, we decide whether to pursue curative treatment and how long to continue in the hospital, running the risk of enduring experiences we may prefer to opt out of. Or, to opt out of the path itself, and die in PEACE in a humane environment under nurturing conditions.

Or, we can choose in advance, coming to grips with our ultimate demise, and coming to peace with the rest of our lives.

Do you want a hospital to be the last place you inhabit on earth?

I imagine that the bravery required to choose against hospitalization (or rehospitalization), to choose to die in PEACE, is among the most heroic actions anyone can take. For those wanting to live the value of individualism completely, choosing against institutionalized dying makes intrinsic sense.

Contemplating Our Own Passing

One element in accepting death is contemplation. Here, I mean contemplation in the deeper sense used by spiritual and religious pursuits. Although not Buddhist, I became aware of one contemplative practice during my attendance at the 2007 Naropa caregiving conference: a short daily meditation on one's own demise, imagining oneself dying and dead. Other religions may have similar contemplative tools. The point is to gain some level of comfort around dying and equanimity with one's own eventual demise.

Perhaps with a fuller understanding of what institutionalized dying entails, an appreciation of all that hospice offers, a reframe of heroism, and some personal work around mortality, we may gain broader equanimity than we have today.

Disenfranchisement and Apparent Opportunity

Earlier, I mentioned that people of color share a concern that the system devalues their lives compared to the lives of white people.

Around Thanksgiving 2006, I listened to a public radio segment discussing how the African-American families interviewed insisted on using the medical system to its fullest during an elder's terminal hospitalization.[104] The idea of abandoning curative treatment was off the table. Consequently, these elders' deaths were prolonged.

The reasons given by those interviewed for their approach ranged from satisfying religious requirements regarding the sanctity of life to the notion of finally being able to insist upon and obtain services from the system, and that doing so compensated, in part, for a lifetime of disenfranchisement.

I cannot put myself in the shoes of Black Americans, or others who are, in feeling or fact, disenfranchised; who may view the unlimited use of medical technology at end of life as an overdue payment of a social debt. Having experienced what I have, I can offer this:

Be sure that the goal of treatment is congruent with your loved one's desires for their end days. Clarify your own patient-family's deepest wishes for how you leave one another in this lifetime. Understand the risks and requirements of terminal hospitalization. Make sure that if you choose to endure the risks, you do so for personally valid reasons that you can look back on without regret.

It's Up to Us: the Imperative for PEACE is Personal

I DID NOT BEGIN THIS BOOK AS AN END-OF-LIFE REFORMER. I became one as the natural outgrowth of my research, analysis, and contemplation.

As a young man, I came to realize that change occurs when continuing to do the same thing becomes more painful than change itself is perceived to be. *Notes from the Waiting Room* has cataloged a range of ways in which hospitalized dying is more painful than the fact of dying need be for many American patient-families. The thought of our citizenry queuing up for these experiences represents more pain on a national scale than is naturally present in dying and death. Any loss due to death is painful. An extended hospitalization experience does not mitigate the loss. The conditions of extended hospitalization we've explored in this book add to the pain, both in real time and in our memories.

Some public policy professionals have wrestled with end-of-life issues for decades. The few times they've gone public has caused a furor. Former Colorado Governor Richard Lamm initiated a national uproar in 1984 with a philosophical reference to the terminally ill having a "duty to die" for the greater social good. In his recent book, *Condition Critical: A New Moral Vision for Health Care*, Lamm presents a well-developed case for end-of-life reform. It's based on the potential for national bankruptcy and the need for making millions of medical decisions based on an expanded sense of the public good. (We've already heard about personal bankruptcies due to healthcare costs, and if hospitals jump on the palliative bandwagon, it may be to stave off institutional bankruptcies that could be brought about by trying to serve growing numbers of dying elders under the current medical model, as Baby Boomers reach seventy and beyond). The public good suggests we bring all Americans "under the tent," with the potential trade-off of "thinning the soup."[105] By this, Lamm means that every American ought to have health coverage, and if providing that means that we each potentially have access to less expensive treatment, particularly at end of life, then the trade-off is ethically sound.

Less known is that medical ethicists have also been trying to forge policies for rationing end-of-life care—again, from a standpoint that "pulling all the stops" is unwarranted and just too expensive. Several groups have convened for approximately two years each, and each group has failed to agree on parameters for rationing.[106] Even clinical ethicists—smart, wise, sensitive, and compassionate people—cannot agree on how to parse resources or what constitutes futility.

Not surprisingly, this debate raises hackles among some physicians, for it proposes a modification to (some might say abandonment of) the Hippocratic oath. It certainly challenges the propriety of cradle-to-grave doctor autonomy. *Condition Critical* must be read to understand the global and national political-healthcare milieu in order to begin to weigh in on its proposal.

Lamm's far-ranging thinking does not extend to providing any tool for how individual patient-families might come to terms with the future he envisions. In this respect, what policy analysts offer differs little from what the medical world offers. Each sector focuses on providing what they can within their perceived charter, stopping short of providing practical guidance for the people they serve. The populace is left on its own to make sense of, to begin to accept, what's offered. Since these matters are not part of our national conversation, and atypically part of private conversations, it's little wonder that we patient-families are surprised, shocked, and distressed with our experience of our loved ones' end days and hesitant about contemplating our own.

In any case, policy analysts and ethicists have already been wrestling with the future shape of medical treatment. A possibility exists, at some point in *our* future, that the system will ration "heroic" treatment, probably in favor of the young, middle aged, and people who do not engage in known unhealthy habits such as smoking (as already occurs in England).[107] If and when these policies are enacted, we cannot expect or rely on policy makers to help us come to terms with them; we can expect only to be advised, in one way or another, to buck up and accept the new reality.

Accepting The Option to Die in PEACE as a viable way out of institutionalized dying is something We the People can do ourselves. Doing so requires a new orientation, a new "container." This container is defined by:

- The reality of timed dying in hospitals
- The realization that suicide is by definition moot once we become irreversibly terminal (for example, voluntarily stopping life support in any form including ingesting pills)
- The freedom from moral angst in facing death once we recognize that the true time of heroic action in all our lives has, for many or most of us, occurred—possibly enduring for years—well prior to the onset of our end days (which for some number of us will represent but a few ten-thousandths of our entire lifespan)
- The presence of hospice for help dying non-institutional deaths, and the slow (albeit eventual) growth of palliative medicine as a branch extending hospice and as a subspecialty of curative medicine.

The container will be deepened if and when heroic-to-futile end-of-life medical options become rationed. We can expand to fill some of that "space" through personal equanimity acquired through contemplation, alone and in groups assembling for that purpose.

One seemingly ironic byproduct of looking straight on at death and dying is a greater appreciation for the life we lead and have remaining. Removing social stigma around discussing death acts like communal resuscitation, allowing everyone to breathe easier and live happier.

We are part of the system. The orientation we bring to the table affects how the system functions. If we insist upon palliative care options within institutions and a streamlined pathway that precludes institutionalized dying, the system will accommodate us. *We must start talking.*

In general, if you're one of the Baby Boom generation, and if your parents, aunts, and uncles are alive and want a guaranteed option to die in PEACE, you must begin creating change now. If you're a Boomer, you yourself have between zero-to-forty years to make dying in PEACE viable before you or your spouse, siblings, and cousins need it. If you're a child of a Boomer, you have the same time frame, for you may be your mom or dad's personal representative. Although this outlines the basic chronology, people of any age are at risk for experiencing needless angst during end days.

Our earthly experience is what we know with certainty. As important, perhaps more important than resting in peace—a speculative notion, despite its ubiquity—is *dying in peace.*

The option to die in PEACE can make our end days worth living. Instead of bringing death into life through extended terminal hospitalization, why not bring a little of heaven's imagined peace into our end days? Doing so would be like slowing down when entering the exit ramp, instead of revving the engine and trying to rebuild the transmission on the way up, with parts littering the roadway as your vehicle fails.

A S MY FATHER USED TO EXCLAIM in moments of satisfaction with his lot, bemusement with humanity's foibles, and his delight in sharing life with those he loved…

"*Oh heavenly days!*"

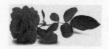

The Option to Die in PEACE Recap: What You Can Do

If your loved one is hospitalized, document everything throughout each day and night. Maintain notes (your personal "chart") or keep a journal.

Be an effective question-asker! *Start now*. Has this chapter answered all your questions about:

- Existing end-of-life options?
- The nature of hospitalized dying and reasons for taking control of our own deaths?
- The Patient Ethical Alternative Care Elective?
- Reframing what constitutes heroic action?
- Coming to terms personally with PEACE?
- Disenfranchisement and apparent opportunity?

If you do not have all the information you need, write your questions down. How will you get them answered? Reread this chapter? Internet research? Library research? Consulting with family and friends? A phone call to a professional or organization? Go online or pick up the phone book, find a likely contact, and send the email or place the call.

SECTION 4 | TOWARD HEAVENLY DAYS

NO MATTER YOUR PROCLIVITIES, bringing a little of heaven's imagined peace into our end days is a valuable personal and societal goal. A peaceful demise makes sense spiritually, ethically, socially, and economically. I propose that we make it our business to make peaceful dying the norm, or at least a normal and supported option. Make viable a pathway to death that embraces dying as the end of human experience, rather than the beginning of a medical melee.

Notes from the Waiting Room postulates that because institutions will be institutions, we as individuals and families must take responsibility for the nature of our end days and how they play out...that a more natural way of dying aided by medical technology for pain relief and comfort will serve everyone involved better than relentless medical intervention in clinical settings.

Fortunately, the institutions may end up joining in this vision by adding to their service model in- and outpatient palliative care services (albeit primarily in response to economic and demographic realities, rather than an innate sense of mission). Until they do, in a manner and to an extent that the majority of hospital-goers receive care—whether curative or terminal—under a palliative umbrella, much needs to change regarding how hospitals and providers function.

Section 4 focuses primarily on steps hospitals and medical providers can take to reform their practice to better humanize their patient-familys' experience.

Chapter 10, "Epilogue and Proposals for Medical System Reform," first closes my father's apartment and my family's personal story, then sets forth numerous suggestions for medical reform.

In suggesting reform I want to acknowledge that physicians and nurses have voluntarily undertaken extensive training (for which they may have accrued substantial debt), and enter demanding professions, through which they attempt to help their fellow humans in direct and often profound ways. Their patient-families form a kaleidoscope of humanity, and they never know which type is going to cross their horizon next. They shoulder responsibilities unknown to many of us.

That said, we will utilize hospitals, even if increasing numbers of us choose not to die in them (a choice not everyone can or will make). We ought not abandon the effort to reform the medical establishment any more than its practitioners (distinct from the insurance industry) would abandon us—even though we would all be better off if the system abandoned dubious notions of what constitutes care, and own up to the realities of what it can and does provide.

In that regard, *Notes from the Waiting Room* concludes with thoughts addressed to medical providers.

10 | Epilogue and Proposals for Medical System Reform

BARELY A MONTH BEFORE FLYING DOWN TO FLORIDA and rushing to my dad's bedside, I spent a week helping him move into his brand-new assisted living apartment. For a total of three weeks during his demise and after his death, I lived in it alone.

That first morning, I entered in the wee hours with the thought that I was merely its temporary caretaker—a story that even then I was afraid I didn't believe. On the bathroom mirror was a post-it note in my dad's scrawl: DRINK WATER. Coming from the Rocky Mountain West, where more than thirty years of arid living has taken a toll on my own hydration, I immediately felt, eerily, that this note to himself was his leave-taking reminder to me.

I tried to minimize the disruption and takeover of my father's space. Nonetheless, each week, my relationship to his space changed. During week one, I rearranged his desk—my new office—and stocked the kitchenette with food to my liking.

As Mort got into deeper water metaphorically, another water metaphor trickled into the apartment. Between hospital visits, a lifelong friend of the family gave me a CD she *liked,* Larger Than Life, *by the Ten Tenors. On it was a waltz-ing ballad, "Water," with the following poignant lyrics:*

> There goes my father
> He's looking at the sky
> He heard of some travellers
> Who make their dreams fly
> I looked into his eyes and saw a river deep and wide,
> He said,
> "I will meet you at the water
> At the water we'll see each other"[108]

During week two, I moved the lamps and the phones to locations in sync with my own movement patterns. By week's end, I'd return from the hospital and continue dismantling Dad's finances and disposing of his property.

I was very aware of my presence amidst a community of elders as I moved about at the quickened pace and purpose of a busy, youthful man. I developed some kind of relation-ship with the men at the widowers' dining table, one of whom I had to remind at each meal just why I was there in my father's seat.

During week three, after Dad's passing, the apartment was my vacant, stripped-down home. I looked out through double windows at the boulevard bordering the grounds, a view Dad had deliberately selected because he liked seeing motion and the human activity it represented. I wondered how future residents might feel, knowing they entered as one among a lineage of elders, people moving into apartments vacated by previous residents who themselves had moved on from this world.

Throughout my stay, I felt gratified at how comfortable an environment Dad had provided for himself after sixty years of married life, and how Deborah had stimulated him to shop with her for some elegant furnishings befitting his new, strange station as a single man.

I donated Dad's newly bought desk with its columns and marble feet to the facility lobby in exchange for a memorial plaque affixed to it. I packed the tool I had made for him just a month before—a large rubber-coated hook screwed into a rod to extend his reach so he could open hallway doors upon scootering straight up to them—a tool now residing above my workbench.

F ROM TIME TO TIME, I'VE BRUSHED AGAINST *what I perceive as the supernatural. Or it's brushed against me. Occasionally, in the wee hours (always the wee hours), I've felt the raised-hair sensation of some presence. During one such instance, I thought, "I can be afraid, or I can not be afraid; why not simply welcome whatever this may be?" Since then, I've chosen to accept the possibility of other-worldliness and view these apparent visitations as neutral and curious, if not benign; perhaps the bearer of some message to be made available upon subsequent reflection.*

Two days after Dad died, a day before my own departure, something strange happened. A reddish-brown drip appeared on the shower wall. It came from beneath the flange holding a grab bar in place, running several inches down the tile. The drip was viscous—definitely not rust-colored water. I had never seen anything like this strange drip anywhere before and have never seen anything like it since.

Despite my penchant for analysis, I opted not to clean it away, nor to remove the flange to investigate this bizarre materialization. I preferred ambiguity. Perhaps, paraphrasing a Rilke sonnet, the drip was a worldly manifestation of Mort's regret.[109] It was then, and remains to me now in memory, a baffling and indecipherable message.

OTHER MESSAGES AND LESSONS RESULTING FROM MY EXPERIENCES during almost six weeks' hospitalization of two dying elders are clearer: extrinsic shocks and their associated angst are not necessary components of dying; diminishing opportunities to commune with and receive direction from a dying loved one can be protected if attention is paid to doing so; the absence of caring support for the patient-family during these most vulnerable times egregiously infringes upon their experience of their loved one's demise; and that caring support is most likely to arise from a non-institutionalized dying environment.

In the introduction, I mentioned that a zillion variables intersect to form the circumstances around each end of life. In a related vein, there are numerous reform initiatives afoot regarding modern medicine. Many of those I've become aware of come from within the bounds of the system's existing functioning. Here are my suggestions, from outside the system, for additional reforms:

Physician Training and Licensure Reform

Require Palliative Training and Licensure for Doctors

Even as palliative medicine is coming into its own as a discipline, every doctor-in-training ought to undergo significant training in palliative care, and state licensure ought to require proven familiarity and competence in palliative treatment, without exception.

Require End-of-life Training and Licensure for Doctors

Death is a part of life, and every doctor ought to be trained in dealing with it. Manifesting a humane orientation around death and the dying ought to be an additional requirement for physician licensure.

Medical students and physicians need to be acculturated differently than in the past, to accept death as the last phase in life. Especially when treating the terminally ill, death ought not be seen as a personal or professional failure. State licensure ought to require a reframe of terminal illness that reflects these points and stimulates subsequent modifications in the role of medicine when attending the dying.

Hospital Administrative Reform

Change How Deaths are Recorded in Hospitals

After doctors are trained to be comfortable with death and licensed to minister to the dying person (distinct from body or component), they ought not be penalized for natural deaths that occur during their attendance when patients remain on a curative treatment path (nor should hospitals be penalized for natural deaths occurring in their facilities). Reporting and recording deaths ought to take into account the circumstances under which they occur, distinguishing deaths from terminal conditions and natural causes from premature deaths, which might rightfully accrue against physician and hospital success ratios.

A special category could track the deaths of individuals who opt to fight until the bitter end. Doctors and institutions assisting those persons could be congratulated for making extraordinary effort (unless we as a society implement a cutoff for expensive, ultra-heroic, futile attempts to forestall dying).

Patient-Family Resources Reform

Employ a Full Team of Ethical Resources in Hospitals

Every hospital ought to have a full contingent of trained professional ethicists on staff and on call for everyone in the institution: staff, providers, and patient-families.

Streamline On-call Ethical Assistance to Patient-Families

Every hospital room and common area ought to have either a call button or Dial H-E-L-P capability for patient-families in distress or decision paralysis to call for ethical assistance. The button or number would ring to either a full-time hospital ethicist-RN or full-time hospital chaplain or mission director.

Patient-Family Treatment Reform

Provide Effective Pain Management

Provider bias and liability impediments to truly effective pain management ought to be removed from healthcare—especially regarding the terminally ill. The technology exists to medically manage pain. It should be available to its fullest potential, directed by the patient, who should be the sole arbiter of appropriate levels and the balance between pain relief and its side effects.

Already proposed by many others is that pain ought to be universally added to the list of vital signs. That list would then read: temperature, pulse, blood pressure, respiration, and pain level. The same approach to fixing or managing the first four vital signs ought to be employed when dealing with pain.

Provide Families 24/7 Access to Loved Ones in ICUs

All intensive care units ought to be open to 24/7 visitation hours. Unless overarching medical reasons exist, family members ought not be excluded from direct patient contact and participation in normal care routines, including touching their loved one. Might this make an ICU staff's job harder? If so, tough—they're not losing a loved one. Might a hospital need more ICU staff? If so, hire them.

Forecast Patient Conditions Continually

Forecasting must be made a non-negotiable, hospital-provider responsibility for every phase of every hospitalization. Advance notice of a range of possible outcomes of short-term treatment and of anticipated choice points' timing and substance should be "SFP": standard functioning procedure. Keeping patient-families in the dark, only to spring pronouncements of the need to make life-and-death decisions as casually as asking if we'd like a mint is *not* good practice. It induces extrinsic shock, delays decision-making, and increases medical expenditures.

Monitor Patients for and Notify Families of the Appearance of Dying Symptoms

Nurses or technicians should be required to monitor for physical and behavioral symptoms that a patient is dying, and notify the family immediately upon observing them. This will require more rounding by hospital personnel.

Due to the potential for patient-families to lose irreplaceable opportunities to commune and to communicate treatment directives, patient-families deserve the earliest possible warning that death may be a real possibility. Notice would be provided immediately when clinically observed conditions known to be associated with dying are first seen.

Provide Complete Disclosure about Resuscitation Matters

Every hospital ought to be required to engage every patient-family in a complete Do-Not-Resuscitate conversation, fully explaining all relevant aspects of resuscitation and DNR status, including sample ethical conundrums and exceptions surrounding its application. The conversation ought to recur as needed as key family members and POAs arrive from afar. Joint Commission accreditation and insurance and government reimbursement ought to hinge on this, and hospitals should require a patient-family signature attesting to having been engaged in the conversation each time. Perhaps the initial "conversation" could occur using a video program, followed by a trained hospital staff member to answer follow-up questions.

Every attending physician should be required to present, in advance of every procedure, their view of their role and responsibilities at the intersection of resuscitation and their direct patient treatment.

Institute Communication Algorithms

Physician-scientists are trained in and use "decision trees" to arrive at diagnoses. The series of if/else questions is referred to as a diagnostic algorithm, a process or set of rules to follow when solving medical problems. Although the best doctors are adept at thinking outside the decision tree to arrive at diagnoses for particularly challenging health problems, the model offers an effective framework for starting many diagnoses.

Accurate communications are as important as accurate diagnoses. All doctors ought to be trained in communication algorithms appropriate to their specialties and be required to prove their competence for licensure.

Communication algorithms should include a range of conversations every specialist can reasonably be expected to engage in based on the nature of their specialty. It should be acknowledged that effective, proactive communication is rightfully the responsibility of the physician (rather than the patient-family), by virtue of their repetitive experience.

Every physician must be capable of engaging in a range of complete conversations that arise as part of their practice. Doctors certainly talk among themselves; why not to the people they serve?

Doctors and ethicists alike have told me that specialists tend to self-select into their medical specialty based on considerations such as personality. Those who don't like talking with customers become anesthesiologists and pathologists, each specialty having progressively less contact with patient-families. Some ethicists propose that they and their fellow ethicists ought to be formally tapped by the system and assigned the role of liaison between patient-families and treatment groups, especially for doctors who may not be comfortable talking at length with their patients. I like this idea of making ethicists available as liaisons. I reject the idea, communicated by one ethicist, that it's either understandable or acceptable for certain specialists to opt out of or be excused from learning and using effective patient-family communication skills. Every physician must be able to communicate outlook and negotiate requirements (both technical and ethical) with their patient-families. I will not excuse unawareness, unwillingness, or inability to do so—my patient-family experienced repetitive harm due to absent communication, at moments representing the crux of each hospitalization/crucible.

One alternative, for doctors who fail communication testing, is a requirement that they arrange for qualified communication surrogates. Ethicists or chaplains could be hired into their practice or arranged for in concert with the hospitals in which they provide services.

Aside from the range of bad news announcements, of particular importance are questions such as:

• What has brought you to this juncture, this decision?

- Would you agree to the recommended treatment if it were approached as a time-based trial?
- What will you do if we do not proceed with what's been medically recommended at this juncture? Will that result be acceptable to you?

When Patient-Families Abandon Treatment, Inquire Why

Any time a patient-family elects to abandon curative treatment and leave the curative hospital jurisdiction, a number of parties ought to inquire as to the reasons. Doing so would not be a thinly veiled effort to prevent the move or persuade the patient-family against moving; rather, the ensuing conversation would be to make certain that no stones have been left unturned. Any conversation would cease upon the refusal of a patient-family to enter into it. The conversation would occur only once and be duly recorded, so that individuals or groups available to function in a safety-net role could be alerted. Thus, other providers would not need to approach the patient-family (and the patient-family would be protected against what they might consider harassment).

I have identified five distinct situations or moments where there was no safety net beneath my patient-family during the DNR snafu that foreclosed Dad's only chance at treatment (his only hope to heal). The first was mine; the other four were institutional or under the purview of providers. They are, in order:

1. My failure to explain Dad's mindset to the anesthesiologists and to tell them that without their agreement, my father would transfer to hospice and die within days.
2. The anesthesiologists failure to completely explain themselves and to inquire into Dad's no-intubation stipulation, uncover his reasons and concerns, and offer potential solutions.
3. The apparent failure of Dad's admitting physician to engage her patient regarding his pending transfer to hospice, uncover his reasons and concerns, and explore alternatives.
4. The hospice's failure to completely examine their prospective patient during intake, unearthing the underlying reason that he presented for admission to hospice.

5. The hospital's failure to investigate, as a matter of patient treatment, why one of their patients had initiated plans to transfer out of the curative environment and enter hospice.

Had an investigative conversation ensued at any one of these missed opportunities, it would likely have brought enough dialog to result in either a time-based-trial approach to Dad's surgery or our *completely educated* refusal of surgery. Four of the five missed opportunities were by the medical establishment, due to disinterest or the absence of formal protocols when life is in the balance.

Place Control Over Dying in The Hands of Those Who are Comfortable With It

Doctors who are uncomfortable with death as the last phase of life and with helping dying people who want to cross over peacefully ought to relinquish control over the dying process. Note that I do not mean for doctors to absent themselves as resources, but to cede control and take a secondary role. Under these circumstances, qualified persons on the palliative care team, including RNs, should have the authority to prescribe pain-relieving medications and their delivery methods without having to refer, or defer, to physicians.

Patient-Family Autonomy Reform

Extend Hospice and Palliative Care Eligibility Forward in Lifetime and Place It Under Individual Control

The Option to Die in PEACE includes a requirement to place eligibility for inclusion within a hospice program (or, looking forward, "roaming" palliative care) squarely into the hands of individuals. The profound shift centers on changing the benchmark from imminent death to something further out on the end-of-life trajectory, replacing a death diagnosis with a clinical evaluation that one's condition more greatly tends toward dying than not, and removing direct physician approval for gaining entry into these programs. We must formalize the understanding that We the People ought to rightfully choose to control our final destiny—not representatives of medical, political, or other establishments.

11 | Thoughts for Medical Providers

I HAVE CRITICIZED INSTITUTIONS for messaging the public with feel-good blather while simultaneously withholding or understating the most vital information patient-families require. Institutions, of course, are made up of both rules and individuals. I spent almost six weeks in two hospitals, in different years and different cities, during two terminal hospitalizations. This string of experiences is sufficient, I believe, to draw conclusions—conclusions that have been verified by a small yet varied sample of healthcare professionals as interviewees and as manuscript readers.

If you recognize the need to have meaningful and timely communication with your patients (customers) but are challenged due to the system, please *just start talking*. I suggest it will ultimately make your job, and everyone's remaining life, easier.

When I say that during hospitalization, the system provides bodily repair services under the direction of independent physician-scientists, do not translate that into an accusation that you are merely a technician. Please do not garble my message, for we both know better. Know that I respect your clinical expertise and the effort it took to obtain and refine it. Own what you do, and if what you do does not map as closely as you'd like to your ideals, modify your service model. In any case, "telling us like it is" would help everybody by alleviating misconceptions. I'd respect institutions and individuals for that candor.

When I say that nurses provide scheduled monitoring rather than care, please know that I assert this with some appreciation of how the system has made nurses' working lives more difficult than ever, and with compassion for what's resulted.

When I expose the gross failure to provide forecasting and the ethical malpractice (as in "bad practice") I believe it represents—based on my family's felt responses to its absence and the irreversible, detrimental consequences which ensued—please take this as a cry in the wilderness to refine your protocols. It's the ethical thing to do.

If you believe in an approach more in line with what I describe as Mom-and-Apple-Pie Care but have reduced your services to something much less, please help to change the system, one patient-family at a time.

T HE RESPONSIBILITY FOR PROBLEMS AND RESOLUTIONS IS SHARED. In my patient-family's cases, I was responsible for not asking all the right questions, for dismissing a patient liaison who may possibly have led us to their answers, and for not completing the communication of our concerns to an anesthesiologist at a critical juncture.

Hospitals were responsible to the extent that they fail to support the family half of their patient-family customers, and for not making clear what family support resources are on staff and exactly how they can help.

Doctors were variously responsible for failing to forecast, failure to attend to a deathbed patient, for not coming clean about or fully explaining reasons for denying patient-family desires, and for neither investigating remaining pathways nor exploring alternatives with the family at a life and death choice point when confronted with a profound, irrevocable decision.

Hospice was responsible for failing to include in its intake process initiatives that would preclude unnecessary family angst, and for failing to investigate the path that led an individual to present himself at hospice, especially when transferring from a hospital bed to a hospice bed just down the hall.

Absent and careless communication detune family functioning like bad air warps musical instruments, resulting in off-kilter harmonics. Since we all breathe the same air, this also makes your job—the entire treatment group's job—here, I'll propose the entire *care team's* job—less... harmonious.

The harm your patient-families experience is not abstract; it interferes with what families most need and value when at their most vulnerable. The issues raised in *Notes from the Waiting Room* beset us during terminal hospitalization. These issues intensify and their consequences worsen during active dying. The harm we endure warps our experiences and resonates, off-key, in our memories.

My compassion for the deep conundrums and stressors healthcare providers face has grown during the years it's taken to complete this book. Nonetheless, if you take a defensive stance in response to the issues I raise, your patient-families will suffer even more extrinsic shocks, adding bitterness to our remembrance of our important time with you. I do not believe that this is what you wish for us, for yourselves, or for the institutions in which you serve.

Afterword | The Moving Medical Target

F ALL 2007: several days after typing the supposedly final period into this manuscript, I learned a few more things.

The venue: a morning panel/discussion hosted by the Denver Community Bioethics Committee, where I met and communed with a palliative care doc who has assumed an administrative role in one of medicine's unique institutions, a hybrid insurer-provider.

During the post-panel reception, Dr. Z suggested that change will occur system-wide and that we'll see it within a decade, because hospitals must respond to the moving medical target, changing demographics, in order to remain solvent.

The situation is this: within ten years, the oldest Boomers will turn seventy and may begin presenting in significant numbers for long-term hospitalizations, including their deaths. They will be covered by Medicare. Since Medicare pays fixed rates rather than open-ended per diems, the financial reality is that hospitals lose money on such patients. Hospitals' prime patients are those who have some procedure and leave within several days. These folks and their insurers pay "full-freight," even if discounted. Revenues from their hospitalizations also pay the difference between what Medicare pays hospitals for the end-of-life crowd and hospitals' true cost of hosting them (cost-shifting, whereby overly profitable business subsidizes money-losing business).

Thus a financial crisis may be brewing for hospitals. How might they resolve it? It turns out that preliminary data shows that palliative treatment delivered by a true team, including physician, ethicist, chaplain, and others, results in improved outcome, improved patient-family satisfaction, and increased profitability. If the metrics hold, the pilot program will run nationwide.

Is Dr. Z's institution well enough respected by the larger hospital systems? Will they notice, and offer their own, patient-family-centric palliative programs? If so, will a deluge of these programs raise all boats, or will they swamp hospice? How will Medicare respond to hospital-sponsored palliative programs in light of its own Medicare Hospice Benefit? How will hospital palliative programs differ from hospice? These are some questions that come to mind.

Even as a slate of new questions arose, an old one got unexpectedly answered. Upon hearing my experiences with hospital communications and that "100 Best" banner, Dr. Z told me what any administrator might have had they taken up my request to discuss why hospitals are the way they are. The answer is tied up in those demographics: hospitals' primary target market is mid-lifers in for short-term (albeit serious and invasive) procedures. Those folks are hospitals' profit center. The banners and happy-couple messages all address them, and are not necessarily meant for the elderly engaged in extended or end-of-life hospitalizations (apparently not even when some of the happy-couple pictures depict the elderly).

I drove home abuzz in an altered state. One previously inexplicable puzzle piece had dropped down, filling a hole in my understanding. I suppose that had I studied business I might have surmised the marketing communication rationale, for every message a business sends has a bottom-line purpose.

As interesting as these demographic revelations may be, they change little if anything at the moment nor, for many of us, for the immediate future. Until palliative care becomes the norm, much will depend upon which doctors attend to each individual during their end of life, whether hospitalized or otherwise. A truly communicative palliative team can offset or prevent transgressions like those my patient-family endured.

Several questions arise from the anticipation: to what degree will the emergence of palliative treatment humanize end-of-life hospitalizations? To what degree will the proposed teamwork comprising palliative care be included with all those non-terminal hospitalizations currently comprising hospitals' profit center? To what extent will palliative teams roam the countryside, becoming the new norm of true end-of-life care?

One hopes all these reforms will happen, and I hope that this book contributes to their development—while in the meantime empowering We the People, as individuals and families, to seize our own end-of-life initiatives before being seized *by* them, so to speak. Doing so is imperative, based on current conditions that moderate my hopeful desire:

- By rights and common sense, all medical treatment ought to fall under the umbrella of palliative care—the raison d'etre for medicine no matter its stripe. As I understand him, Dr. Z's goal is a complete reframe of the current medical paradigm, to ensure that this becomes the case. This is a huge undertaking that requires concurrence and active participation by the nation's hospitals, medical schools, and all its independent physician-scientists.

- Dr. Z's got his work cut out for him as exemplified by commentary in the Journal of the American Medical Association by Robert Holloway MD and Timothy Quill MD[110] (the latter described to me as the father of modern-day palliative medicine). These doctors end their peer commentary with the statement, "...prior research show(s) that patients who are better informed are more inclined to want less aggressive treatment—a strategy that may improve quality while paradoxically increasing mortality." I find nothing at all paradoxical about this combination of conditions. That doctors find it paradoxical underscores this: even the best doctors (defined for our purposes as oriented toward palliative care, hopefully as a norm) seem to remain inside the "box" of allopathic medical thinking, or need to appear that way to their peers. An examination of either conclusion immediately brings to mind a number of questions...

...which I shall not pose in *Notes from the Waiting Room*. Clearly, much reframing remains to be done by all of us when it comes to contemplating, and experiencing, our end days. We will all need to reestablish profound levels of trust:

- Individuals trusting their sense of what's right and appropriate at the end of life, relative to the entirety of their life
- Families members trusting their dying loved ones to know and pursue what's right for themselves
- The medical establishment trusting people who ask for its beneficence while rejecting its remove and control
- Patient-families trusting the medical establishment, and its motives for pursuing comfort versus cure as each case, and palliative options, unfold
- Citizens with differing viewpoints trusting that many truths attend humanity, being willing to leave various pathways open for those who want to walk them.

Perhaps the additional contemplation required to reframe the way things are into the way things could be represents the seed of a sequel to *Notes from the Waiting Room*.

Acknowledgments

I FIRST WANT TO ACKNOWLEDGE Judy Greenberg, my sister, a now-retired newborn intensive care nurse who worked for thirty-five years with newborns, including the prematurely born ("preemies") who fit within her cupped palms. During each of our parents' demise, Judy persevered despite serious medical conditions of her own.

Few of us are fortunate enough to have competent medical practitioners in the family. Judy's ethics regarding patient care are clear and strong, and her clinical knowledge was often relevant to adult care. She knew what medications were being administered, what the machines were signaling, what the staff was (or should have been) doing, and what competent medical care consists of. She also immediately recognized its absence.

Deborah Fink's encouragement, her belief in the value of this effort, and her tolerance of its demands represent twin center poles of support—personal pillars of Asclepius and Caduceus.

Although this book is based primarily on my family's experience, the experiences of other families also informs this discussion. Thanks to those friends, acquaintances, and "plain folk" who shared their stories and insights. I am humbled by their willingness to reenter years-old grief with me. I hope you feel that what I've offered herein justifies the revisited pain of your remembrances.

I am deeply grateful for and to the medical, scholarly, and legal professionals who so generously shared their time, experience, interest in, and encouragement of this book.

I want also to acknowledge providers: those attending to my parents, and providers in general. They work hard, in challenging conditions. Almost to a man and woman, they mean well.

I cannot heap enough gratitude on those comprising my "reader team," who volunteered their time reading the draft manuscript in its awful, unedited, primitive form and who offered spirited and thoughtful feedback: Jeff Brenninger, Jeffrey Duvall, Bob Eaton, Deborah Fink, Nick Gatel, Judy Greenberg, Rhy Jouett, Michelle King, Carol Sheer,

Doug Smith, Mary Ann Strobridge, and Diann Uustal. Each of you are in this book through the suggestions you offered for its improvement.

Thia Rose early on pointed me in the right research direction, opening what became a cascade of interviewees without whom I could not have completed this work.

A bow is due my editor, Jasmin Cori, who helped sculpt *Notes from the Waiting Room* into cohesive form. Through the editing process, this first-time author came to learn that the manuscript brought forth over several years was more raw than I had believed it to be. Jasmin prompted me to untangle my thoughts on both small and large scales by directly challenging my confused writing, and by modeling clearer thinking.

Here's appreciation for Paul Shippee, who in 1993 suggested I investigate the story of Orpheus as a gateway to writing an article for the Underworld issue of the (since-defunct) *Mens Council Journal*. Besides finding a wickedly delightful tale of the Muse, the inquiry yielded Rilke's masterwork, with which I was then unfamiliar. That I found it in the form of Steven Mitchell's translation was pure good fortune. This lineage is the foundation of my profound moments in Eldorado Canyon.

Thanks, too, to the Colorado Independent Publishers Association and its membership for countless learning opportunities. CIPA is a mature, robust, proactive group with practical wisdom that I have gratefully tapped.

Copywriter and author Peter Bowerman helped identify and refine the too-elusive title, plus the exact wording of the subtitle and sub-subtitle, bringing to bear his especially keen linguistic discernment.

Kudos to, and gratitude for, George Foster for creating a strong yet sensitive cover, balancing and finessing more communicative design elements than many covers require, and for incorporating this ex-pro designer's proclivities. Working *with* top pros (distinct from hiring them) is exhilarating.

Brian Allen and Ronnie Moore each cast their expert eyes on the nearly complete layout, offering perceptive suggestions to enhance its beauty and readability respectively, which I have done my best to incorporate. Any impurities remaining accrue from my sole sensibilities.

Marilyn Anderson's perceptive indexing and Bonnie Beach's sharp-eyed proofreading helped neatly tuck the book together in its final stages. I claim full responsibility for any remaining loose threads, e.g., content anomalies.

Lastly, I acknowledge you, the reader. These topics are among the most challenging, and I thank you for joining me in a commitment to examine them in the light of day, for it's time to reform end of life in our society before the hours grow dark for each of us.

AND OF COURSE I ACKNOWLEDGE MY PARENTS, Morton and Ruth Hanna Logue Greenberg. I dedicate this book and The Option to Die in PEACE to their memory. Perhaps one of the most important lessons we can learn from our parents is to not make the same mistakes they have made. My parents' lives, interwoven through a marriage of more than sixty years, were right for them. As a middle-aged son and father, I periodically examine their choices and map my own against them.

Ultimately, this book is about learning *how* to choose *what* to choose, especially when faced with events causing us to contemplate and accept our own, and our loved ones', mortality.

To Mort and Ruth, I say, rest in peace.

To the rest of us, I add, rest in *PEACE*.

D<small>URING MY RESEARCH,</small> I <small>EXAMINED A VARIETY OF BOOKS</small> to one degree or another. I had two goals. First, to learn as much as I could absorb, particularly from those works relevant to my research. Second, to determine if I could find anyone who had already written the things I've been saying (with the partial exception of Mark Meaney, no one was or has).

The following short list presents the books I found indispensable in understanding why things are the way they are when we die in hospitals, what to do about it, plus some interesting books on related matters. These are the books I read cover to cover and made part of my physical or mental library.

The Best of the Best

T<small>HE FIRST TWO OF THE</small> "<small>BEST BOOKS</small>" provide the most vital on-the-scene assistance every personal representative must have and know. Interestingly, and like *Notes from the Waiting Room*, they either are or were originally published by companies their authors founded. Each is somewhat idiosyncratic, revealing a little more of their authors' personality than sometimes comes across in books polished by traditional major publishers. The practical information each book offers is easy to find.

These two books are essential. I will carry and refer to them during my next family hospitalization, and have directed my family to do likewise if that hospitalization is mine. Keep their essential pages with you during any hospitalization:

Hospital Stay Handbook: A Guide to Becoming a Patient Advocate for Your Loved Ones by Jari Holland Buck (Llewellen Publications, 2007)

Originally published as *24/7 or Dead* (AuthorHouse, 2006), this is the ultimate field manual for personal representatives. Buck, a layperson, writes an authoritative personal account of managing life-threatening hospitalizations. Her previously healthy, middle-aged husband (a lawyer who did not execute any Power Documents for himself and his family) would have died without her involvement as his personal representative. *Hospital Stay Handbook* underscores the notion that the real potential for serious problems exists at any hospital, even those at the top tiers with the highest reputations. Contains various checklists indispensable for personal representatives, including criteria for assessing different types of facilities. *24/7* was a quick, easy read/reference, perfect for keeping with you 24/7 when hospitalized. Hospital Stay Handbook almost doubles in size, adding Buck's considerable spiritual experience to the mix.

3 Secrets Hospitals Don't Want You To Know: How to Empower Patients by Mark Meaney (NIPR Press, 2006)

Meaney's insider status as a hospital ethicist is refreshingly used to present street-smart, practical guidance for patient-families in the crucible of problematic hospitalizations. At this writing, and so far as I know, Meaney and I are the only people who comprehensively describe how to find and obtain on-site ethical assistance when conflicts arise during hospitalizations. Meaney's inclusion of historical policy benchmarks adds stature to *3 Secrets*. If you need to go the ethical distance with surety, you'll want *3 Secrets* as a reference. Keep it in your pocket.[111]

THE FOLLOWING BOOKS ARE USEFUL TO ALL, providing the factual and cognitive framework for taking control of our own dying:

...And a Time to Die: How American Hospitals Shape the End of Life by Sharon Kaufman (Scribner, 2005)

...And a Time to Die is a mind opener. It documents Kaufman's two-year research project examining hospitalized dying in America. Kaufman, a professor of medical anthropology, was the ultimate fly on the treatment group wall. Stay with her lengthy examination and case studies, and the gravity of her insights will reward you (the rewards actually start early on). This work absolutely reshaped my outlook about morality and autonomy at end of life, as it may yours. Its revelations represent one pillar supporting acceptance of The Option to Die in PEACE.

Patient-Directed Dying: A Call for Legalized Aid to the Dying for the Terminally Ill by Tom Preston, M.D. (iUniverse Star, 2007)

Reframing unexamined beliefs is the foundation for solving gnarly ethical-medical problems. Preston reframes what "terminal" means and what follows from that, logically and ethically, when people become terminal. *Patient-Directed Dying* joins ...*And a Time to Die* as an intellectual and moral bookend around the justification (if not imperative) to control one's own end days. Preston's reframe represents the second pillar supporting how to accept The Option to Die in PEACE.[112]

Last Rights: Rescuing the End of Life from the Medical System by Stephen P. Kiernan (St. Martin's Press, 2006)

Kiernan, an award-winning healthcare journalist, has assembled an impressive extended reportage examining how end of life has changed during our lifetimes. As befitting the work of a journalist, *Last Rights* presents numerous facts interwoven with analysis and commentary. *Last Rights* is enriching, bolstering the imperative to act to reform end-of-life options. With its delicacy of thought and expression, this elegant, captivating work is a vital addition to that imperative.

Condition Critical: A New Moral Vision for Health Care by Richard D. Lamm and Robert H. Blank (Fulcrum Publishing, 2007)

Former three-term Colorado Governor Richard Lamm has long advocated for systemic healthcare reform from his unique perspective as a state's chief executive officer. In this policy essay, Lamm expands his long-held viewpoint that in some instances (including end of life), curative medical intervention ought to be withheld. Lamm and Blank articulate a future of rationed care based upon the simple fiscal unsustainability of "blank check" medicine where doctors are the arbiters, although other parties (including future generations) pay the bills.

Unsustainable costs inform the distinction between the health of society versus the health (and health choices) of individuals. What makes this book so relevant to *Notes from the Waiting Room* is its vision of healthcare rationing policies that would, in effect, prompt members of the Boomer generation into PEACE or PEACE-like dying scenarios.

The Rest of the Best

THE NEXT GROUP OF BOOKS ARE ALL BY DOCTORS. Explanations from physicians and surgeons themselves are always valuable, as much for what they don't say as what they do. I always hope for insiders to bust out of the boundaries defining their professional world, even though that's almost always asking too much, for they don't. This is vital to know, because it underscores that We the People have a necessary and legitimate role to play in taking control of our end days. By doing so, we also help physicians, who benefit from the relief as much as we do, even though they may not yet feel comfortable telling us so.

Final Exam: A Surgeon's Reflections on Mortality by Pauline Chen (Knopf, 2007)

Finally, the opportunity to learn the surgeon's side of hospitalization, dying, and death. Unique and refreshing in its openness, this book comes from a member of a group that this layperson could not break into to engage in conversation. Chen discusses some of what lay people may have surmised about surgeons based on their own transitory contact during hospitalizations. She's articulate, insightful, and actually does share a surgeon's unique viewpoints. Hallelujah for Chen's humanity.

You: The Smart Patient by Michael Roizen, Mehmet Oz, and The Joint Commission (Free Press, 2006)

This witty book had me wondering who the ghostwriter is. *You: The Smart Patient* is a clever offering, cloaking a potpourri of serious information in the costume of levity. You'll smile a lot, which is a good thing. The problem with this book is that, while it presents itself as a complete compendium of insider information, it doesn't cover the major topics in *Notes from the Waiting Room*. In a way, I don't mind.

How to Get Out of the Hospital Alive by Sheldon Blau, M.D. and Elaine Shimberg (Macmillon, 1997)

A full-of-facts book about managing hospitalization that offers nitty-gritty information. That Blau is a doctor who suffered surprise heart surgery lends credibility to this offering.

How We Die: Reflections on Life's Final Chapter **by Sherwin Nuland, M.D. (Vintage, 1995)**

How We Die describes in detail how the various major diseases causing death play out. This is useful, if difficult, information to know.

Dying Well: Peace and Possibilities at the End of Life **by Ira Byock, M.D. (Riverhead Books, 1997)**

Through stories, Dr. Byock compassionately shares his insights into reforming end of life. Contemplative in nature, the stories, as ever, incline one to mutely acknowledge the work we may have to do to die in peace. Byock, now an end-of-life reform icon, seems to have accepted early on the role that contemplation plays during the end days.

To Die Well: Your Right to Comfort, Calm, and Choice in the Last Days of Life, **by Sidney Wanzer, M.D. and Joseph Glenmullen, M.D., (Da Capo Press, 2007)**

To Die Well presents a cogent case for hastening death. For those so inclined or interested, this book is a valuable examination and guide.

THE FOLLOWING BOOKS ARE EXCELLENT RESOURCES on topics closely related to managing hospitalization and end of life. Practical or quirky, these topics are streams we enter when following the overflowing waters of the metaphorical pond. Let the waters flow.

Grave Matters: A Journey Through the Modern Funeral Industry to a Natural Way of Burial **by Mark Harris (Scribner, 2007)**

One thing leads to another. Those who opt out of hospitalized dying may also decide to opt out of delayed and prolonged decomposition and the exorbitant fees paid to accomplish it. *Grave Matters* exposes how things work and what options we have to depart from a previously unexamined mainstream. Harris examines all manner of traditional and alternative funeral and burial options. Contact information is included throughout for readers to acquire state-specific information and other needed resources.

Stiff: The Curious Lives of Human Cadavers by Mary Roach (W. W. Norton and Company, 2004)

Roach's offbeat topic fascinates completely, as does her voice. Her writing is a hoot. While almost totally tangential to the real-life problems associated with hospitalization and dying, if you're intellectually inclined to breathe life (or at least utility) back into the dead, *Stiff* reveals the many uses to which human remains can be, and are, put.

The Sonnets to Orpheus, Rainer Maria Rilke, Translated by Stephen Mitchell (Simon and Schuster, 1985)

Rilke, among the twentieth century's preeminent poets, brings us as close to the mysteries of death as is earthly imaginable. His genius is exquisitely matched by the genius and elegance of Stephen Mitchell's translation, where the right word exposes the unexposeable, expresses the unsayable, just as the right facet reveals a diamond's complete beauty: again and again and again, and again, eternally.

THIS BOOK IS USEFUL FOR UNDERSTANDING what hospitals have been through the ages:

Mending Bodies, Saving Souls: A History of Hospitals by Guenter Risse (Oxford University Press, 1999)

I referred to this scholarly tome as part of my quest to understand, if only a little, the whats, whys, and wherefores of hospitals as institutions. *Mending Bodies, Saving Souls* is a rich look at hospitals through the millennia, from which we can take as little or as much as is possible for a mind to absorb. Good for perspective, decidedly not required scanning (let alone reading).

Endnotes

Thoughts for Those in Acute Need or Crisis

1   Angel: a particularly wise, sensitive, and compassionate doctor, nurse, or ethicist with enough time at that moment to give you conclusive assistance and support.

New Terms for a Clear Conversation

2   *Last Rights: Rescuing the End of Life from the Medical System*, Stephen Kiernan, St. Martin's Press, 2006.

3   Healing is another word used by two constituencies. Medicine uses "healing "to describe its clinical activities. Healthcare reformists use "healing" to describe what they consider to be more humane, compassionate actions and approaches addressing aspects of patients' humanity that modern medicine in large part ignores.

4   An example of when ethical assistance might be required is if the treatment group and patient-family cannot agree on the parameters for providing (or ceasing) treatment or the extent to which to treat.

5   By this I mean that hospitals as institutions do not provide care. As you'll read, even many individuals who work within hospitals (employed or independent) do not provide care. Occasionally, an individual doctor or nurse does provide caring attention. In our experiences over about 6 weeks, these moments were few, neither frequent nor sustained enough to change the overall troublesome nature of each hospitalization.

6   Estate settlement is the subject of my companion book, *How to Efficiently Settle the Family Estate*, Axiom Action, 2007, which is downloadable from www.AxiomAction.com.

7   Attributed to the clinical ethicist Diann Uustal, RN, MS, Ed.D.

8   Ibid.

9   DNRs are executed by physicians on behalf of patients. Typically only the very infirm and/or elderly will possess a DNR (by contrast, anyone can and should execute a Living Will).

10   An un-word is a word currently in use but not yet formally acknowledged as a word by its inclusion in a major, recognized dictionary.

11   Medicine distinguishes between the dying process in general and *active dying*, the latter indicating the duration of the final physical shutdown leading up to the moment of death.

Preface | The Genesis of Notes from the Waiting Room

12   Medical anthropology: the study of humankind in the medical environment.

13   More so for my companion book, *How to Efficiently Settle the Family Estate*, Axiom Action, 2007; downloadable from www.AxiomAction.com

14   Executive management model: an organizational scheme whereby a cadre of high-level peers are replaced by a smaller number of hierarchical executives and a larger number of lesser-paid workers whose roles are narrow when compared to the cadre they replace.

15   In real life (distinct from television), doctors and nurses refer to the Emergency Department or ED. If I occasionally use "ER" (for emergency room) it's because the rest of us so commonly use it.

16   The sole exception I'm aware of is the appearance in early 2007 of Mark Meaney's book, *3 Secrets Hospitals Don't Want You to Know*, now one of my top three recommended resources.

17   Health treatment providers may challenge this assertion. My experience and research reveal instances in which applied life-support technology is viewed by clinicians as a form of treatment rather than life support. This can become a catch-22 should disagreements arise between treatment providers and the patient-family regarding details of, or limitations on, a course of treatment.

18   Dad was in shock; his partner of sixty years was dying (1) unexpectedly and (2) everyone had thought she would outlive him.

19   Somewhere in my research (I don't recall where), I came across a statement that the most typical occurrence regarding family members is that a middle-aged son shows up midway through a terminal hospitalization. Then, regardless of an advance directive and whatever relationship other family members may have established with the treatment group, he begins directing the show, frequently according to his own worldview rather than the loved one's. This may, in part, explain why providers would tend to address me rather than Dad (given his infirmities). The compassionate viewpoint is that providers need our help in remembering who their primary family member or medical POA may be—*especially if it's the elderly spouse.*

20   From my perspective, the only reason to have left monitoring equipment hooked up to our dying mother was for the nurses' *convenience* (yet the alarms were ignored when they did ring out). To be fair, the plan was to move Mom into hospice; she just didn't make it that long and wound up dying in the ICU about 7 hours after extubation. For dying loved ones coming off life support, arrange for hospice intake in advance and leave life support in place until transfer to hospice can coincide with life-support removal. This will increase the chance that your loved one's end hours and your experience of them are reasonably humane.

Introduction

21   Some healthcare policy analysts, such as former Colorado Governor Richard Lamm, foresee national bankruptcy unless bold steps are taken immediately.

1 | Be an Effective Personal Representative

22 According to Dad, he had designed the first color television kit for home assembly. Electronic do-it-yourself kits were all the rage among guys fascinated with the then-new video and audio offerings of the mid-twentieth century (when Radio Shack was solely the ultimate geek heaven).

23 The Medical Durable Power of Attorney document is one of a suite of core legal documents I call "Power Documents." These are described in the Power Documents chapter.

24 This is known as "incapacity" and requires two physicians' signatures.

25 State laws play a formal part and vary from state to state.

26 Insofar as financial concerns may impact medical treatment, a property power of attorney is important to set up. Primarily, though, property and financial concerns arise when settling a family estate.

27 HIPAA: the Health Insurance Portability and Privacy Act protecting individuals' medical information.

28 See *Hospital Stay Handbook* by Jari Holland Buck, Llewellen Publications, 2007.

29 Recent reports suggest that cell phones do not interfere with hospital equipment. Citation: The Mayo Clinic, March 8, 2007.

2 | Making Effective Declarations: The Essential Power Documents

30 Health Insurance Portability and Accountability Act.

31 My lawyer provided me with blank signature pages for all of my family's POAs for us to execute on our own each year.

32 Again, see *Hospital Stay Handbook* by Jari Holland Buck, Llewellen Publications, 2007.

33 Crash: a term really used in healthcare, designating a sudden, serious health failure.

34 Technically, the body's cells continue living for some hours after what we recognize as death has occurred. According to Joan Halifax Roshi during Naropa University's 2007 *Integrating Spirit & Caregiving Conference*, a future technological level regarding resuscitation may well be the cellular. At some point, what we recognize today as death may be subject to revision. Today, we can resuscitate people within a short time after heart or breath has stopped; in the future, the time during which resuscitation is possible may elongate. In any case, ongoing cellular life may present an interesting subject of contemplation for philosophers and ethicists.

35 Wills, trusts, and effective estate settlement are topics of the companion book to *Notes from the Waiting Room, How to Efficiently Settle the Family Estate*, Bart Windrum, Axiom Action, 2007. Downloadable from www.AxiomAction.com.

36 The relative cost of having a last will and a trust drafted equates to dropping several quarters in a parking meter versus paying a $50 fine (and loosing access to your car until the fine is paid and has cleared the bank).

3 | Differing Sensibilities: Care and Communication in Hospitals

37   Not to be confused with the Caduceus, the emblem of two snakes entwined around a staff with a pair of wings atop the staff of commerce.

38   According to Judy Greenberg, RN (NICU), due to the growth of patient care centers that are independent of hospitals, the trend is for patients of traditional hospitals as a group to be sicker than previously. Thus, hospital nurses' patient loads are more likely to include more very ill patients.

39   Medical mistakes are the focus of some Joint Commission reform efforts and the subject of repeated popular media coverage.

40   Faith-based hospitals' operations are informed, in part, by their religious mission and hence have mission departments, under which pastoral and ethical support services are provided and managed.

41   A series of charts succinctly summarize differences between various types of hospitals, but requires deciphering due to confusing formatting (at least in the initial version, *24/7 or Dead*).

42   A relatively new type of hospital is the physician-owned facility. These range from small units providing specialized services (example: colonoscopy) to full-sized hospitals. Carefully investigate the policies of and staffing provided by such institutions, which may not have any doctor in-house on weekends.

4 | Family Involvement in Hospital Care

43   What would turn out to be an agonizingly painful wrist infection immobilized his right hand. His left arm was bound up with multiple IVs.

44   Judith Briles, *Zapping Conflict in the Health Care Workplace*, Mile High Press, 2003, 2008.

45   MRSA: Methicillin-resistant Staphylococcus Aureus, an extremely antibiotic-resistant infection common in hospitals today. Treatment requires Vancomycin, a particularly strong antibiotic that shows signs of becoming ineffective in fighting the infection. In elders, serious illness can result from infection, including pneumonia.

46   Most hospitals request that cell phones be turned off in the halls and units on the grounds that they interfere with the functioning of bedside machines. One recent study asserts that cell phones do not interfere with bedside machinery (although they do interfere with certain diagnostic equipment). It could be that we'll see a general relaxing in the policy that asks us to turn cell phones off. As a practical matter, you may find it difficult to manage the hospitalization if having to rely on hospital telephones alone.

47   To be fair, part of a nurse's role is to relay doctor comments and actions to the family. Attentive nursing care is crucial to good patient-family care. Yet it does not substitute for face time with the doctors on your loved one's case, especially when trying to prepare the family for whatever comes next.

48   Acquiring ethical assistance in the hospital (if it is available) is discussed in chapter 7, "The Complete Do-Not-Resuscitate Conversation." Assuming a mature ethical environment, lawsuits may be very avoidable by engaging the help of the pastoral care department and the on-site help a chaplain can engage on your behalf.

49   These conferences were the genesis of my investigation into the nature and reality of hospital communication, representing this book's inception. I just didn't know it at the time.

5 | Forecasting and Ethical Support: What You Need to Know, When You Need to Know It, and How to Get It

50   I came close to crying at that moment, despite experiencing a profound sense of relief. Holy smokes, our cumulative experiences had a *name*! However unfortunate the fact that these experiences were common enough to have earned a name, the *acknowledgment* implicit in this name, "forecasting," was profound, for it identified what was denied us throughout both terminal hospitalizations.

51   According to one source, less known is that the directive to "act for the good of [patients]" appears before the more widely known dictum to "first do no harm." These related phrases combine to form a more powerful statement than either alone.

52   That's what it *felt like* at the time. With the benefit of more than two years' inquiry, evaluation, and epiphany, I have come to realize that while we might have believed we held Dad's life in our hands, the overarching likelihood was that his life was over. Faced with the imminent loss of a loved one, it takes a different type of being than mine to free our perceptions during such times. Perhaps a non-human being. The problems stem from a misperception of what occurs during the end days, when multiple levels of experience overlap, forming a sort of gravitational force from which it is impossible to escape into clarity and lightness. These levels include emotions, ethics, medical prerogatives, spirituality, religion, attachment, the law, politics, command/control imperatives, and perhaps simple inertia.

53   "We Forecast Early and Often" ought to be a creed for every hospital. In practice, we don't get to choose which hospital we enter. Emergencies and health insurance plan requirements play a large role in determining which hospital many patients are admitted to.

54   *3 Secrets Hospitals Don't Want You to Know: How to Empower Patients*, Mark E. Meaney, NIPR Press, 2007 (a must-carry book for any hospitalization).

55   Some hospitals may employ one or more full-time chaplains and utilize rotating chaplains during off-hours.

56   Do these questions seem off-putting? Perhaps more gracious people than I can restate them or preface them with a statement such as "please forgive me, but I must ask you several very direct questions." In any case, their essence remains. These are the most serious issues occurring during the most traumatic of times. There is no room, nor need, for tiptoeing around the interface of treatment, care, advocacy, and outcome when your loved one's life is at risk.

6 | Who's Where, When, Why, for How Long, and Other Turns through the Hospital Maze

57   Bodily distress can be readily observed, for example shivering, grimacing, fluids in the endotracheal tube.

58   I've read an anecdote about specialists rounding at four or five a.m., getting troubling findings, and prescribing drugs to counteract them. This is likely a strange exception, but let's address it anyway. The problem with pre-dawn examinations has to do with lack of patient responsiveness due to their metabolism being low (it's the wee hours). Check with the doctors about their rounding times, and if something like this comes up, discuss your concerns with them.

59   See my companion book *How to Efficiently Settle the Family Estate* for discussion of many aspects of and situations encountered during estate settlement. Axiom Action, 2007; downloadable from www.AxiomAction.com.

60   Compliments of the U.S.-Iraq war comes the phrase "Improvised Explosive Device."

7 | The Complete Do Not Resuscitate Conversation

61   Current statistics report that only 15% of Americans have completed an advance directive.

62   Schiavo's was not the first such case to reach national attention, but it was the first to end up with the U.S. Congress passing legislation focused directly and only on it in an attempt to intervene.

63   First responders are typically fire department personnel trained as EMTs, Emergency Medical Technicians.

64   Defibrillation is the introduction of electric shock to restore a regular heartbeat, usually by "paddles."

65   An invasive medical procedure is one in which something penetrates into the body through the skin or a cavity.

66   See *Final Exam: A Surgeon's Reflections on Mortality*, Pauline W. Chen, Alfred A. Knopf, 2007.

67   Finding the Emanuel questionnaire may be difficult, as the work was part of an academic study. Ask your nurses and doctors if you're interested in obtaining this or something like it.

68   According to unnamed studies cited in *Last Rights: Rescuing End of Life From the Medical System* (Stephen Kiernan, St. Martin's Press, 2006), the percentages fall on the low end of the ranges. Dr. D suggests that those numbers could be doubled or tripled and fall with his anecdotal experience; hence the range I use.

In either case, the percentages of people within and outside of hospitals who survive resuscitation, let alone return to full functionality, appear very small.

69   This assumes that you do not feel that death is the worst possible outcome.

70   An old U.S. Army acronym—Situation Normal All Fucked Up—now generally accepted as "a confused state" (Apple Computer Dictionary v1.0.1 application under Mac OS X).

71   Catheterization relieves the need to urinate into a bedpan, directing the flow instead into a bag hanging on the bedside.

72   Heart attack.

73   I am fully aware that death due to arrest can be reversed. Does this make sense for the very infirm elderly? For each of us, our own morals must guide.

74   When I ran this claim past my primary ethical interviewee, she suggested we might be surprised at the number of college students who are under DNR status due to grave medical problems.

75   "The Science of Death: Reviving the Dead," Jerry Adler, Newsweek July 23, 2007.

76   It's been known for many years that organs continue living for some time after a time of death has been declared.

77   To familiarize yourself with the institutional lineage of patient's rights, I highly recommend Dr. Mark Meaney's short and authoritative book, *3 Secrets Hospitals Don't Want You to Know: How to Empower Patients*, NIPR Press, 2007.

8 | Death Looks Like This

78   Plastination is the progressive replacement of bodily fluids with substances that essentially plasticize the body. This preserves the body in a remarkable state. Museum exhibitions containing dozens of plastinated bodies tour the globe. See www.BodyWorlds.com.

79   For discussion of conventional and green burial options see *Grave Matters*, Mark Harris, Scribner, 2007. For discussion of the various scientific uses to which corpses are put see *Stiff: The Curious Lives of Human Cadavers*, Mary Roach, W. W. Norton and Company, 2004.

80   One notable exception is the film, *The Three Burials of Melquiades Estrada*, Sony Pictures Classics, 2005.

81   A situation that has since changed: the facility's executive director said that within the past several years, "many" of their assisted living residents had died in their apartments, including those who had left for the hospital and returned from it to die at home. She suggested that they disallowed residents' dying at home for some time immediately after opening the facility to minimize the complications that resident deaths would present until they smoothed out operations. This was an understandable but unfortunate stance, and represents another question to ask of any assisted living facility your loved one may consider for residence.

82   See *Grave Matters* (endnote 79) for good documentation on how to manage the disposition of remains, depending upon the conditions of death and the type of treatment you plan.

83   Ibid.

84   See my companion book, downloadable from www.AxiomAction.com: *How to Efficiently Settle the Family Estate*, Bart Windrum, Axiom Action, 2007.

85   First read *Grave Matters* and follow the guidance provided. See each of its chapter's end pages for listings of resources.

9 | The Option to Die in Peace: Patient Ethical Alternative Care Elective

86   Rainer Maria Rilke, *The Sonnets to Orpheus*, sonnet II:XIII.

87   According to a hospital chaplain in my community whose hospital has pioneered a palliative care program, inquiries from other hospitals for doing so have increased during 2006 from a handful to significantly more than he can respond to.

88   It's important to distinguish between plain straight talk among a dying loved one, the POA, and family members from the use of metaphor as a poetic way to understand one's world. I employ metaphor in this book to help us understand our experiences. At the bedside, as events unfold in real time, metaphor cannot substitute for clarity of speech and thought. Once clarity of *intention* has been established and reality recognized with no embellishment, metaphor can be useful to help make sense out of what seems senseless, if that's your style.

89   Many private insurance policies have a hospice benefit, so check yours carefully.

90   Despite a hospice demise costing about half as much as a hospitalized one.

91   End stage: the very end of end of life, known in medicine as "active dying."

92   More than one of my medical professional manuscript readers has told me that doctors confide in them that, in many instances, they are relieved when their patient-families conclude that death is inevitable and are prepared to "allow" their loved one to die. Anecdotes in some of my suggested reading mention nurses privately confiding that the treatment group is often collectively relieved when a patient-family assents that it's time to let go.

93   Kaufman cites various examples of patient-families receiving mixed messages from treatment group members.

94   I submitted an early version of The Option to Die in PEACE as a health care reform proposal to the 2008 Colorado Blue Ribbon Commission for Health Care Reform, convened by the Colorado state legislature in early 2007.

95   Subject to whatever future modifications to treatment procedures may be in effect. For an interesting conversation about healthcare rationing, see *Condition Critical: A New Moral Vision for Health Care*, Richard Lamm, Fulcrum Publications, 2007.

96   Note that the risk of a partial loss of dignity and control exists for anyone experiencing physical breakdown. For some, dying will be messy. Loss of physical control is a real privation, but the overall loss of control is exacerbated when the patient-family is removed from a private home and must conform to the rules, operation, and values of some institution.

97   *Patient-Directed Dying: A Call for Legalized Aid in Dying for the Terminally Ill*, Tom Preston, M.D., iUniverse Star, 2007.

98   An interesting aside: what would it take to round out that $7/100^{th}$ of one percent to $1/10^{th}$ of one percent, i.e., $1/1000^{th}$, or the last $1/1000^{th}$ after $999/1000^{th}$ of one's lifespan? Assuming a terminal hospitalization of 3 weeks, it would take a lifespan of approximately 58 years. Before running the calculation, I had thought the age would dip only slightly, from 80–85 years to about 75. I think most of us would agree that, absent restrictions, a 58 year old in medical crisis represents a life with enough future potential (12–25 years) to spare no effort in saving—putting the patient-family firmly into the crucible of a no-holds-barred hospitalization.

99   Proportionality is the fourth condition inside the Principle of Double Effect (attributed to the thirteenth-century theologian, Thomas Aquinas). It's a baseline of ethical decision-making during end of life. Proportionality says that the good result of a decision must be proportionate to any attendant bad result in order for the bad result to be acceptable.

100   When I described this hypothetical situation to one medical ethicist, she suggested that it could easily fail, that many doctors would order a psychological evaluation and that the process could drag on for 30, 60, 90 days. The result would have been Dad languishing at home for longer than he might have wanted or succumbing to a hospitalized death in the interim. On the other hand, hospice programs exist to serve people in their own choices. Deciding against eating pills is an individual right, and a good hospice program would, after ensuring that their patient was mindful of where such a pathway leads, proceed to do what they always do—keep the dying comfortable and at peace.

101   I encountered several at a Naropa University 2007 caregiver conference.

102   I suspect caregiver stress syndrome as one cause of my mother's demise.

103   Heroicism: conduct or behavior relating to heroism; a lesser form of heroism. (www.unwords.com)

104   An article also addresses this issue: "At the End of Life: A Racial Divide," *Washington Post*, March 12, 2007.

105   From an interview with Governor Lamm on *Colorado Matters*, August 14, 2007, Colorado Public Radio.

106   (1) Reuters News Service, "Death and Dying: When is it Time to Let Go?," retrieved from www.CNN.com August, 2007; (2) personal conversation with Diann Uustal, clinical ethicist.

107   *Condition Critical: A New Moral Vision for Health Care,* Richard D. Lamm and Robert H. Blank, Fulcrum Publishing, 2007.

10 | Epilogue and Proposals for Medical System Reform

108 "Water/Va Pensiero," *Larger Than Life*, The Ten Tenors; Richard Vella, lyricist. Rhino Records, 2004. Used by permission of Richard Vella.

109 Rainer Maria Rilke, Sonnet II:XIV, Stephen Mitchell translation: "perhaps it is our vocation to be their regret."

Afterword

110 *Mortality as a Measure of Quality: Implications for Palliative and End-of-Life Care*, Robert G. Holloway, MD, MPH and Timothy E. Quill, MD, Journal of the American Medical Association (JAMA), August 15, 2007, Vol 298, No. 7

Recommended Reading

111 Had I had *3 Secrets* during my father's 2005 hospitalization, it's likely that the book you're holding would not exist, because our problems might have gotten solved. Mark and I were amazed to learn that we both address how to find ethical support in hospitals, not exactly a common topic in hospital self-help books (actually, as of this writing, it's a topic unique to *3 Secrets* and *Notes from the Waiting Room*).

112 The third pillar is my own offering, the reframe of what constitutes heroicism.

Index

Note: Italics denote references to the family anecdotes, which are also italicized in the text. Endnotes are denoted by an "n" following the page number. Multiple notes are denoted by "nn."

A

Abandonment
concept, 257, 316n92
of treatment
questioning why, 289–90
requirement for hospice, 252
Acceptance of death, 239, 253, 316n91
Accessibility of documentation, 92
Action, empowerment for/urgency for, 53
Acute
defined, 144
effects of extrinsic shock, 143–44
Acute need or crisis, thoughts for those in, xiv–xviii
avoiding terminal hospitalization, 243–44
death looks like this, 219–40
forecasting and ethical support, 139–141
hospital maze, 162–64
hospitals, care and communication in, 101–3
Option to Die in PEACE, 243–44
personal representative, 60–61
Power Documents, 79–80
providing care in hospital, 119–20
resuscitation/Do Not Resuscitate (DNR), 183–84
Administration, hospital. *See* **Hospital administration**
Advance directives, 25, 86
need for, 64–65
See also Living Will; Medical Durable Power of Attorney
Agent, for Power Documents, 26, 62, 83, 91
Agonal respiration, 236

Algorithms
communication, 287—289
diagnostic, 287
Allopathic physicians, 268, 317n101
American Medical Association, palliative medicine subspecialty, 246
...And a Time to Die **(Kaufman),** 255, 304
Anecdotes. *See* **Family anecdotes**
Anesthesia, general, DNR order and, 194, 199–201
Asclepius, 103, 312n37
Assisted dying, 248
See also Patient-directed dying; Self-directed dying
At-home (unattended) deaths, 236–37, 316n82
Authentication, defined, 27
Author (Bart Windrum)
background, 32, 39
blame, not motivation for text, 37–38
companion book on Estate Settlement, 309n6, 316n84
disclaimers, 39
dissatisfaction clarified, 40–41, 40–43
genesis of book, 29–43
patient liaison, contacts during father's hospitalization, 157, 201, 202
personal representative role, 74
research beginnings, 31–32
theses, 36–37
Author's family
stories/case studies/recollections. *See* Family anecdotes

B

Baby Boom generation, 276, 295
Bankruptcy, national, 274
Banners as billboards, 110–11
Beliefs, identifying, 264–65, 317n99
Bias, medical, 267
Blanket, need for, 100
Bodily repair services, 104–7, 291
Body after death. *See* **Corpses;
     Death looks like this**
Buck, Jari Holland, 108
Burial options, 224, 315n79

C

Caduceus, 312n37
Cancer, terminal diagnosis, 248–49
Cardio infarction (heart attack),
     200, 201, 315n72
**Cardiopulmonary resuscitation
     (CPR),** 189, 191
   implied consent for 911 calls,
      195–96
   no-CPR directive, 89
Care, 22, 108–16, 309n5
   caregiver stress, 69, 317n102
   defining, 103-4, 108–09
   discontinuity of, 22, 129–31
   in hospitals, 52–53, 108–16
      pastoral care, 36–37
      provision by family, 126–27
      recap, 116
   as human endeavor, 105
   Mom-and-Apple-Pie, 109, 121, 292
   our understanding vs. medical
      establishment's, 105
   taking care of yourself, 61 71
   why we expect care from hospitals,
      108–13
   See also Treatment
Caregiver stress syndrome, 71,
     317n102
Care team. *See* **Treatment group**
Case manager, 154
Catheterization, 198–199, 315n71

Cell phones, 70, 311n29, 312n46
Certification of death, 237
Certified Nursing Assistant (CNA),
     167
Chaplain, 139–41, 154–56, 285,
     313n55
   author's interviews with, 35–36
   defined, 154
   as expert communicator, 155
   first question to ask, 155
   forecasting/ethical assistance and,
      154–56
Charge Nurse, 168
Chart
   hospital, access to, 69, 311n28
   medical, flagging of DNR on, 183,
      193
   personal representative's, 69
   See also Medical records
Chemical life support, 38, 137–38
Chen, Pauline, 265, 304
Clinical ethicists, 36
   See also Ethics
Closest relative, 82
Code Blue, 191
Code/coded, 191
Coma, 236
Communication, 52–53, 99–16, 291,
     292–93
   absent and careless, 292–93
   algorithms, 287–89
   discontinuity of, 129–31, 133
   "don't ask, don't tell" norm, 72
   in hospitals, 108–16
   as intrinsic part of care, 103–4
   lost opportunities for, 176
   Patient's Bill of Rights and, 72
   poor, extrinsic shock and, 37
   recap, 116
   self-serving, by hospitals, 109–13
   significance of, 103–4
   what we really need to know from
      hospitals, 115–16
   who is/should be addressed, 41,
      310n19

See also Communion; Hospitals, care and communication in
Communion, 220
   defined, 24–25
   lost opportunities for, 176, 245
Communities, home-like, dying in, 268–69
Complaints (who not to complain to), 131–34
Condition Critical **(Lamm and Blank),** 273–74, 305–6, 317nn105-6
Confusion, 234
Control
   of eligibility for hospice/palliative care, 290
   loss of, 260
   reforms suggested, 290
   taking control. *See* Option to Die in PEACE
   transferring, 267–68
   See also Option to Die in PEACE
Corporatization of hospitals, 122–24
Corpses
   father's remains, 223–25
   handling the body, 236–37, 316n82
   spirituality and, 225–26
   uses for, 224, 315n79
   viewing the remains, 226–27
   See also Death looks like this
Cost shifting, 254
CPR. *See* **Cardiopulmonary resuscitation (CPR)**
Crash, medical, 87, 271, 311nn33
Cremation, 238
Crisis. *See* **Acute need or crisis, thoughts for those in**
Crucible
   defined, 71
   end-of-life experiences as, 175–77, 246–47
   as heart-warming opportunity, 170
   hospitalization as, 175–77, 246–47
   personal representative role as, 71
   as 7 ten-thousandths of lifespan, 263–64, 317n98

D
Death
   accepting, 239, 253, 316n91
   ambivalence about, 255
   behavioral symptoms of, 234–35
   beliefs about, 264–65
   biological, 89, 311n34
   certification of, 237
   contemplating our own, 272
   denial of, 227
   factual description of, 223–25
   fear of, 261
   finality of, 223
   hospital categories for, need for new, 285
   hospitalized, nature of, 254–58
   hospitals, managed and timed in 256–58
   media depictions of, 227–28, 315n80
   medical bias against, 267
   natural, 262
   options, need for new, 254
   options for, existing, 248–54
   recording of, by hospitals, 285
   signals of, 231–33
   symptoms of impending, 233–36
   uncompromising reality of, 220
   versus demise, 27
   See also Death looks like this; Dying; Option to Die in PEACE
Death certificates, 237
Death looks like this, 219–40, 239
   accepting death, 239, 253, 316n91
   arrangements for body after death, 236–37, 316n82
   at-home (unattended) deaths, 236–37, 316n82
   behavioral symptoms of impending death, 234–35
   burial options, 224, 315n79
   certification of death, 237
   changing our experience of death, 239
   conditions you may encounter, 226–27

conversations not held with parents, 228–31

death certificates, 237

depiction, importance of accuracy in, 222–23

depictions by media, 227–28, 315n80

finality of death, 223

funeral arrangements, 238–39, 316n85

handling the body, 236–37, 316n82

mortuaries, 237, 238–39

physical symptoms of impending death, 236

picking the air, 232–33, 235

pre-need contracts, 238, 239

recap, 239–40

remains of father (Mort), 223–25

signals death may be near, 231–33

spirituality and corpses, 225–26

symptoms of impending death, 233–36

symptoms of impending death, monitoring for, 287

uses for body, post-death, 224, 315n79

viewing the remains, 226–27

See also Death; Dying

Death rattle, 236

Declarations, effective, 77–79

See also Power Documents

Defibrillation, 189, 193, 314n64

Definitions, 19–27

Delays in hospitals, 164

Delusions, 235

Demise, defined, 27

Digital voice recorder, 69–70

Dignity, loss of, 260, 317n96

Disability insurance, 135

Discharge from hospital, financial concerns, 123

Discontinuity of care, 22, 129–31

Discontinuity of communication, 129–31

Disenfranchisement, 272–73, 317n104

DNR. See **Do Not Resuscitate (DNR) conversation**

Doctors

admitting, 172

author's interviews with, 34

communication among, 129–30, 312–13n47

communication reforms suggested for, 287–89

communication with, 128–31

firing, issues to consider, 170, 174–75

as hospitalists, 131, 147, 169

orders, delays in implementing, 164

presence/absence of, 165–66

residents, 168–69

responsibility for problems, 292

rounds, hours of, 41, 147, 164–65, 314n58

thoughts for, 291–93

training and licensure, reforms suggested for, 284

who performs surgery?, 168–69

See also Independent physician-scientists

Documentation

of conversations, observations, actions, 68–69

original versus copies, 92

power document accessibility, 92

Power Documents, 77–94

Do no harm principle, See **First do no harm**

Do Not Resuscitate (DNR) conversation, 97, 179–212, 287

Code/Full Code/Code Blue, 191

conclusion and recommendations, 210–12

definitions, 189–90

DNR

active status, requirements for, 185–86, 190–91

cardiac DNR, 197

conditional DNR, 197

emergency/first responders and, 92, 190, 195–96, 314n63
   questions to ask, 186–87, 193
   treatment goals and, 187–89, 205-6
DNR bracelet/medallion, 89, 195
DNR directive, 185, 189, 190
DNR form, 88–89, 190
   accessibility of, 92
   definition of, 189–90
   differences from Living Will, 190
   differences in forms of, 194–95
   hospital's non-revocable DNR, 195
   "refrigerator" DNR, 195
   submission at hospital admission, 186
DNR order, 53, 189, 190
   actions of (when a DNR is in effect), 190
   college students with, 209, 315n74
   consequences of not having, 192–93
   definition of, 190
   denial as matter of policy?, 208–09
   flagging on medical chart, 183, 191
   non-recognition of in-effect order, 193–94
   permanence of, 194
   recission during surgery, 194, 199–201, 207
   time to take effect, 191
DNR snafus, 196–201, 287–88, 315n70
   snafus #1 and #2, 179–83, 197–198
   snafu #3 (operate or die), 198–201, 205–08, 263, 289–90
DNR status
   emergency/first responders and, 79, 92, 195–96, 314n63
   verifying, 192–93

when is DNR in effect?, 185–86, 190–91, 193
ethical gray zones, 184, 196–209
   DNR snafus, 197–203
   doctor interpretation, 198
   ethical slicing and dicing, 201–3, 206
   intersection of provider viewpoints and resuscitation, 204–08
   operate or die (snafu #3), 198–201
911 calls, 195–96
recap, 212
recommendations, 210–12
resuscitation, 52–53, 88–89, 187–96, 311n34
   effectiveness of, 196, 314–15n68
   ethical gray zones, 196–209
   future choices, 209–10, 315nn75–6
   practicalities and legalities, 189–96
   treatment goals and, 187–89
   unexpected circumstances, 197–201
"Don't ask, don't tell," 72, 211
Double effect, principle of, 264, 317n99
Durability, power of attorney, 83
Dying
   active, 309n11
   assisted, 248
   due to "wrong turn," 249–50
   fear of, 261
   at home, in home-like communities, or hospice, 268–69
   medical bias against, 267
   non-institutionalized, 26–27
   patient-directed, 262–63, 265, 317n97
   process of. *See* Demise
   self-directed, 248–49
   symptoms of, monitoring for, 287
   See also Death; Death looks like this
Dying Well (Byock), 307

E

Effective, defined, 57

Emanuel, Linda, 194, 314n67

Emergency department (ED), 96
  emergency room (ER), 96, 310n15
    doctors, author's interviews
      with, 34
  experiences intensified in, 106–7

Emergency responders. *See* **First responders**

Emergency room (ER), *See* **Emergency Department (ED)**

Emotional understanding, 53, 95

End-of-life
  existing options, 248–54
  hospitalization, present technol-
    ogy/times and, 113–14
  imperative to change, 215–17
  rights, 32
  training, 284
  See also Death looks like this;
    Option to Die in PEACE

Entity/entities
  dealing with, 46–47
  defined, 27

Epilogue, 281–97

ER. *See* **Emergency room (ER)**

Estate settlement, 23
  death certificates for, 237
  estate value and, 90
  *How to Efficiently Settle the Family
    Estate* (Windrum), 309n6,
    316n84

Ethical assistance, 21, 97, 203, 309n4
  asking for/need to ask, 152
  ethics committee, 156
  hospital chaplain, 154–56, 285
  hospital Mission departments, 285,
    312n40
  obtaining, 52–53
  on-call assistance, 285
  patient liaison/patient advocate,
    152–54
    case manager, 154
    registered nurse (RN), 153–54
    social worker, 153
  specialist liaison, 153
  printed materials, 152
  recap, 158
  reforms suggested for, 285
  registered nurse (RN), 153–54
  resolving conflicts with treatment
    groups, 151–51
  summary, 157–58
  support for forecasting, 149–56

Ethics
  ethical environment, 151–53, 156
  ethical gray zones, 184, 196–209
  ethics committee, 35, 156
  "first do no harm" principle, 114,
    142, 200, 204, 313n51
  healthcare rationing and, 274,
    317n106
  medical ethicists, 36, 131, 274
  medical ethics, 32, 141, 144, 194,
    201
  See also Ethical assistance

Euthanasia, 248

Executive management model, 32,
  310n14

Expectations, 108

Experiences behind this book,
  29–30

Extrinsic shock. *See* **Shock**

Extubation, 179–80, 205

F

Families, 117–36
  defining, 51–53
  family-focused medical environ-
    ment, 149–50
  family-friendly hospital environ-
    ment, 127–28, 146, 150
  information needed from hospi-
    tals, 115–16
  insurance issues, 134–36
  involvement in hospital care, 97,
    101, 117–36, 144
  large, need for advance directives,
    64–65

locations for treatment discussions/conferences, 128–30
need to oversee treatment, 126
percent capable of managing hospitalization/death, 106–7
provision of care in hospital, 126–27
recap, 138
support services, hospital, 146
who not to complain to, 131–34
who pays and how much, 134–36
who to talk to, 129–31
See also Patient-family
Family anecdotes
agonizing decisions over medications, 146–47, 313n52
author's reflections on mother's terminal diagnosis, 241–42, 316n86
conversation Dad and I didn't have, 228–30
conversation Mom and I didn't have, 230–31
father, walking out, 203–4
father, diminished self-restraint, 235
father, operate or die/DNR snafu #3, 198–201
father, peaceful demise: example not manifested, 266–67, 317n100
father, picking the air, 232–33
father calls a "meeting", 57–59
father not eating in hospital/family-paid assistance, 117–18, 312n43
father's deathbed, 219
father's hospice entry/discontinuity of communication, 159–61
father's hospital admission, 77–79
father's recovery visualized/expected by author, 202–3
father's remains, 225
hospice intake/forecasting, 137–38
mother's ICU stay/DNR and extrinsic shocks, 179–82
mother's ICU stay/engaging nursing management, 131–33
mother's ICU stay/low body temperature, 99–100

night my father died, 17–18
"Oh heavenly days," father's expression, 276
water metaphor/brush with supernatural, 283
water metaphor/living in Dad's apartment, 281–82
Fears, identifying and overcoming, 260–62
Final Exam (Chen), 265, 306
Financial Power of Attorney. *See* **Property (financial) Durable Power of Attorney**
Financial professionals, author's interviews with, 33
Firing nurses, doctors, and hospitals, 170–75
"First do no harm," 114, 144, 200, 204, 313n51
First responders, 79, 92, 195–96, 314n63
need to see DNR form, 190, 195
Forecasting, 52–53, 97, 137–58, 205, 286, 313n50
asking for/need to ask, 152
back-end, 148–49
defined, 23–24, 141–42
ethical support services to assist, 149–56
ethics committee, 156
final comments, 149, 313n53
front-end questions to ask, 146–48
hospital chaplain, 154–56
how to recognize, 72
patient liaison/patient advocate, 152–54
case manager, 154
registered nurse (RN), 153–54
social worker, 152
specialist liaison, 153
printed materials, 152
recap, 158
shock due to lack of, 139, 142, 144–45, 199, 201, 290
significance of, 141–49
summary, 157–58

using the term, 144
versus prognosis, 144, 144–46
"We Forecast Early and Often," 149
See also Ethical assistance
Full Code, 192
Funeral arrangements, 238–39,
    316n85
Funeral home. *See* **Mortuary**
Funeral professionals, author's
    interviews with, 32
Futility, concept of, 270

G
Genesis of this book, 29–43
Grave Matters **(Harris),** 307
Gray zone of indetermination, 255
Gray zones, ethical, 186, 198–21111
Grief, 29–30

H
Hallucinations, 235
Headset, for cell phone, 72
Healing, 23, 107, 309n3
Health care rationing, 274–75,
    316n95, 317nn106-7
Healthcare system
    as broken, 51, 310n21
    changing, 51
    opting out of, 51
    understanding, 48–49
    See also Option to Die in PEACE
Heart attack (cardio infarction),
    202, 203, 315n72
Heavenly days
    father's expression, 276
    moving toward, 279–80
Heroic action/heroics. *See* **Heroicism**
Heroicism, 269–73, 318n112
    contemplating our own passing,
    272
    defined, 29, 317n103
    description of, 269
    disenfranchisement/racial issues,
    272–73, 317n104

in father's last 19 years, 271
futility, concept of, 270
prior to terminal hospitalization,
    270–72
redefining, 269–73
resuscitation for elderly/infirm as,
    192
HIPAA (Health Insurance Portability
    and Accountability Act), 25
HIPAA Authorization and Release
    document, 69, 85–86
    submission at hospital admission,
    185
Hippocratic oath, 250, 274
Home, dying at, 268–69
Hospice, 251–54, 269
    abandonment of curative treat-
    ment required, 252
    advance planning for, 310n20
    cost of, 251, 252, 316n90
    cost shifting and, 254
    differences in, 254
    eligibility, current, 251–52
    eligibility, reforms suggested for,
    290
    hospice entry/second consult requested
    (father), 159–60
    hospice intake (father), 137–39
    insurance and, 251, 316n89
    intake nurse fired (father's), 173–74
    leaving/reentry, 252
    pain management, 248–49
    palliative care in, 251–52
    pre-hospice consult, 213
    responsibility for problems, 292
    as station of last resort, 253–54
    terminal diagnosis required, 252
Hospital administration
    hospital administrators, defined,
    35
    nursing management, 131–34,
    167–69
    reform of, 285
    thoughts for, 292
Hospital-borne infections, 125,
    312n45

Hospitalists, 131, 147, 169
Hospitalization
  as a crucible, 177–79
  alternatives to, 37
  characteristics experienced, 106
  effectively managing, 95–97
  hospitalized dying, cost of, 268
  list of questions for, 146–48
  Power Documents and, 81
  problems experienced by author
    and family, 40–43
  problems with, 37
  risks of, 119, 125–26
    breaches of hygiene, 125
    hospital-borne infections, 125,
      312n45
    mislabeled IV fluids and
      medications, 126
  See also Option to Die in PEACE
Hospital maze, 97, 159–78
  calendar considerations/days of
    week, 166
  coping (if all else fails), 176–77
  doctors, presence/absence of,
    165–66
  doctors' rounds, hours of, 41, 147,
    164, 165–66, 314n58
  firing nurses/doctors/hospitals,
    169–75
  hospitalization as a crucible,
    175–77
  Hospital Time, 148, 162, 164–66
  insurance concerns, 175
  multiracial environment, 169–70
  recap, 177–79
  who administers to your loved
    one?, 167–70
  See also Hospitalization; Hospitals
Hospitals, 99–116
  accreditation, 212
  admission
    forms to submit, 185–86
    verifying DNR status, 192–93
  bodily repair services in, 104–7,
    291

  care/communication in. *See*
    Hospitals, care and communica-
    tion in
  causes of present conditions/status,
    121–25
  changes over time, 121–23
  corporatization of, 122–24
  death managed and timed in,
    256–58
  delays in, 164
  differences in, 108, 312n41
  discharge from, 123
  family-focused medical environ-
    ment, 149–50
  family-friendly environment, 127–
    28, 146, 150
  family involvement in care, 97,
    101, 117–36, 144
  financial crisis brewing for, 295–96
  firing issues, 174–75
  Hospital Time, 148, 162, 164–66
  "hundred best," 110–11, 117, 127
  insurance and treatment goals,
    122–23
  leaving, procedure for, 174–75
  locations of treatment discussions/
    conferences, 128–29
  Mission Statement, 111
  morgue in, 237–38
  as multiracial environments,
    169–70
  non-provision of care, 31, 36–37
  nursing care, 105, 123–24, 312n38
  opting out of terminal care/treat-
    ment. *See* Option to Die in
    PEACE
  Patient's Rights placard, 111–12
  physician-owned, 312n42
  redefining, 20, 104–7
  religiously based, 155, 312n40
  responsibility for problems, 292
  services provided, 96
  training/skill level of staff, 167–70
  types, comparison of, 107–8
  what we really need to know from,
    115–16

See also Hospitalization; Hospital
   maze
**Hospitals, care and communication
   in,** 96–98, 99–106
   banners as billboards, 110–11
   brochures and handbooks, 112–13
   family involvement in, 97, 101,
      117–36, 144
   lobby placards, 111–12
   naiveté in expectations?, 108–9,
      113
   non-provision of care, 31, 36–37
   print advertisements and website
      images, 112
   recap, 116
   redefining hospitals, 20, 104–7
   redefining the patient, 113–15
   self-serving communication,
      109–13
   significance of communication,
      103–4
   what hospitals communicate,
      109–13
   what we need to know, 115–16
   why we expect care, 108–13
***Hospital Stay Handbook* (Buck),** 108,
   303–4
Hospital Time, 148, 162, 164–66
***How to Efficiently Settle the Family
   Estate* (Windrum),** 309n6,
   316n84
***How to Get Out of the Hospital Alive*
   (Blau),** 308
***How We Die* (Nuland),** 309
"Hundred best" hospitals, 108–9,
   115 125
Hygiene, hospital breaches of, 125

I
ICU. *See* **Intensive care unit (ICU)**
**Identification, of IV fluids and
   medications,** 126
Imperative to act, 53
Incapacity, 62, 311n24
   power of attorney and, 83

Independent physician-scientists
   bodily repair services from, 105–7,
      291
   communication among, 129–30,
      312–13n47
   communication reforms suggested,
      287–89
   communication with, 128–31,
      312–13n47
   defined, 21
   thoughts for, 291–93
   See also Doctors
Infections, hospital-borne, 125,
   312n45
Informed consent, 206, 209
Insurance, 134–36
   disability, 135
   DNR conversation and, 287
   end-of-life issues concerning pro-
      gression/regression, 257
   "gap" insurance, 134–35
   hospice and, 251, 316n89
   hospital choice/leaving a hospital,
      175
   hospital treatment goals and,
      123–24
   Medicaid, 135
   Medicare, 134, 135, 251
   pre-existing conditions, 135
   private, 135
   who pays and how much, 134–36
Intensive care unit (ICU)
   access to loved ones, reform sug-
      gested, 286
   firing considered, 174–75
   mother, ICU experience, 174–75
   *mother's stay, DNR and extrinsic
      shocks,* 179–83, 197
   *mother's stay, engaging nursing man-
      agement,* 131–33
   mother's stay, low body temperature,
      99–100, 103
Intrinsic shock. *See* **Shock**
Intubation, 184, 189, 205–8
   alternatives/alternate scenarios,
      203–4, 207–8

extubation, 205
refusal to operate without, 199–201, 206–8
See also Do Not Resuscitate (DNR) conversation; Resuscitation
Invasive, defined, 314n65
Invasive mechanized breathing apparatus, 189
IV fluids, mislabeled, 126

J

Joint Commission, The (TJC), 212
accreditation, DNR conversation and, 287
hospital hygiene, 127
"hundred best" hospitals, 110–11, 117, 127
Journal, personal representative's, 69
"Juice"/unjuiced story, 31–32

K

Kaufman, Sharon, 32, 254–58
Kiernan, Stephen, 32, 267

L

Lamm, Richard, 273–74, 317n106
Laryngeal Mask Airway, 208
Last Rights (Kiernan), 32, 267, 305
Last Will and Testament, 90, 312n36
See also Living Will
Lawsuits, 131, 313n48
Lawyers
author's interviews with, 33
availability/schedule of, 166
elder medical-financial specialty, 135–37
location within residence jurisdiction, 83
for Power Documents, 82, 91, 93
size of law firm, 93
Legislation, for PEACE alternative, 259, 316n94

Licensing, physician, reforms suggested for, 284
Life support, 38, 255, 310n17
chemical, 38, 137–38
guidance in Living Will, 90
Living Will, 25, 86–88
accessibility of documentation, 92
adding Medical POA contents to, 86
DNR form, differences from, 190, 194–95
DNR statement/directive in, 189, 190
issues to consider, 87–88
renewal/re-execution of, 88
submission at hospital admission, 185
versus Last Will and Testament, 86
versus Medical Power of Attorney, 88
Lobby placards, 111–12
Lost opportunities, 176, 245

M

"Machine" terminology, 245
Malpractice, 95
shock due to absence of forecasting as, 144, 292
Meaney, Mark, 32, 155
Media depictions of death, 227–28, 315n80
Medicaid, 135, 212
See also Insurance
Medical anthropology, 32, 309n12
Medical bias, overcoming, 267
Medical chart. *See* Chart
Medical Durable Power of Attorney. *See* **Power of Attorney**
Medical ethicists, 36, 131
healthcare rationing, policy development, 274, 317n106
Medical ethics, 32, 144, 201
forecasting and, 141
non-recognition of DNR as breach of, 194

See also Ethics

Medical mistakes, 106, 312n39

non-recognition of DNR as, 194

Medical providers, thoughts for, 291–93

Medical records

access to, 69, 311n28

HIPAA Authorization and Release and, 69, 85–86

Medical Power of Attorney and, 87–88, 311n32

See also Chart

Medical system reform. *See* **Reform**

Medicare, 134, 135, 212

hospice benefit, 251

See also Insurance

Medications, mislabeled, 126

Mending Bodies, Saving Souls **(Risse),** 308

Metaphors

author's use of, 316n88

as a way of understanding the world, 316n88

canyon as death state, 241–42

crucible, end-of-life experiences as, 71, 175–77, 246–47

father's crude metaphor, 58

getting the weight off, 216

heroicism as crucible, 269–70

metaphorical pond, end-of-life navigation/tossing waters, 246–47

metaphorical pond, Rilke's sonnets/Eldorado Canyon, 241–42, 247

metaphorical pond, ripples in, 49–50

metaphorical stone/renewing cycle, 232

water, as life-death, 242, 247

water, Ten Tenors, 282

water metaphor/brush with supernatural, 283–84

water metaphor/living in Dad's apartment, 281–83

Mislabeled IV fluids and medications, 126

Mistakes, medical, 106, 194, 312n39

Mistreatment, father's inflamed wrist and, 171–72

Mom-and-Apple-Pie care, 109, 121, 292

Morgue, hospital, 237–38

Morphine patches, 248–49

Mortuary, 237, 238–39

MRSA, 125, 312n45

N

Naiveté of expectations, questioned, 101, 108–9, 113

Naropa University Conference (2007), 269, 272, 317n101

National Institute of Medicine, 212

Netherlands, assisted dying in, 248

New terms, 19–27

911 calls, 195–96

No-CPR directive, 89

Non-institutionalized dying, defined, 26–27

Nurses

author's interviews with, 33

Charge Nurse, 168

as communication/information resource, 130, 312–13n47

firing, 170, 171–74

Licensed Practical/Licensed Vocational Nurse (LPN/LVN), 167

Registered Nurse (RN), 153–55, 167

RN as patient liaison/advocate, 153–54

thoughts for, 292

training/skill levels, 167

See also Nursing care; Nursing management

Nurse's Aide (Certified Nursing Assistant/CNA), 167

Nursing care

caseloads, 123

corporatization of hospitals and, 123–25

as hospitals' primary mission, 105, 312n38

production-line model, 123–24

question on gaps in, 147

reduced patient contact, 124

responses to stress, 124, 312n44

sicker patients and, 124–25

Nursing management

complaining to, 131–35

positions/duties, 167–69

O

Operate or die snafu, 198–201, 205–8, 263, 289–90

Option to Die in PEACE, 26, 241–77

as a choice, 259

contemplating our own passing, 272

cost of hospitalized dying, 268

definition of terms in PEACE acronym, 258–59

disenfranchisement/racial issues, 272–73, 317n104

dying at home, in home-like communities, or hospice, 268–69

eligibility to die in PEACE, 259–60, 290

existing end-of-life options, 248–54

dying expectedly due to "wrong turn," 249–50

dying in a planned manner, 248–49

dying under palliative care, 250–51

euthanasia, assisted dying, or self-directed dying, 248–49

hospice, 251–54

sudden natural or accidental death, 248

suicide, 248

fears, identifying and overcoming, 260–62

fear of death, 261–62

fear of dying, 261

fear of losing dignity and control, 260, 317n96

fear of pain, 261

heroic action, reframing, 269–73

hospitalized death, nature of, 254–58

abandonment concept, 257, 316n92

death brought into life, 255–56

gray zone of indetermination, 255

management and active timing of deaths, 256–58

moving things along, 257, 316n93

identifying your beliefs, 264–65, 317n99

medical bias, overcoming, 267

natural death, 262

patient-directed dying, 262–63, 265, 317n97

peaceful demise example, 265–66, 317n100

PEACE (Patient Ethical Alternative Care Elective), 258–59

imperative for, 273–76

need for, 254

overcoming obstacles to, 260–69

recap, 276–77

7 ten-thousandths, 263–64, 317n98

the system, we are part of, 275

taking control of our deaths, 258–60

transferring control, 267–68

Oregon, assisted dying in, 248

P

Pain

fear of, 261

as fifth vital sign, 251, 286

management in hospice, 248–49

management under palliative care, 250–51
morphine patches for, 248–49
relief, addiction and, 250–51, 261
relief, loss of consciousness and, 250
Palliative care, 246, 250–51, 316n87
addiction and, 250–51
allopathic physicians and, 268, 317n101
definition of palliative, 250
eligibility, reforms suggested for, 290
future of, 250, 295–298
loss of cognition and, 250
outside of hospitals (Option to Die in PEACE), 258–59
palliative care team, 252
training for doctors, 284
Palliative medicine, 246, 284
Pastoral care personnel, author's interviews with, 35–37
Patient. See Patient-family
Patient advocate, 23, 114, 152–53, 157
need for, 126, 144
See also Personal representative
Patient-directed dying, 262–63, 265, 317n97
Patient-Directed Dying (Preston), 32, 305
Patient Ethical Alternative Care Elective (PEACE). See Option to Die in PEACE
Patient-family
defined, 21
family provision of care, 126–27
oversight of treatment, 127
redefining the patient, 113–15
resources, reforms suggested for, 285
treatment, reforms suggested for, 286–90
See also Personal representative; Reform
Patient liaison, 23, 139, 152–53

author contacted during father's hospitalization, 157, 201, 202
author's interviews with, 33
See also Personal representative
Patient representative. See Personal representative
Patient rights, 32, 171, 315n77
hospital Patient's Rights placard, 111–12
Patient's Bill of Rights, 72
PEACE (Patient Ethical Alternative Care Elective). See Option to Die in PEACE
Personal representative, 57–76
cell phone for, 70, 311n29
as champion of loved one's wishes, 63–65
defined, 22–23
designation as, 62
documentation/records, 68–70
effectiveness, aspects of, 63–71
effectiveness, defined, 55
family benefits of, 73–74
financial representation, 65
functions of, 62–63
importance of, 72–75
information needed from hospitals, 115–16
journal of, 69
legal interpretation of, 30
need for, 63
personal "chart" of, 69
for Power Documents, 62, 83, 91
question-asker role, 65–68, 72–73, 74–75
recap, 76
taking care of yourself, 71
tape or digital voice recorder for, 69–70
time demands on, 70–71, 73
who not to complain to, 131–34
who to talk to, 139–31
See also Power Documents
Physicians. See Doctors; Independent physician-scientists

Picking the air, 232–33, 235
Plain folk, 33
Planned dying, 248–49
Plastinization, 224, 315n78
Power Documents, 77–94
  acceptable documentation, 92–93
  acceptance, state laws and, 82–83
  accessibility of documentation, 92
  agent/personal representative des-
    ignation, 62, 83, 91
  consequences of having or not
    having, 81–82
  defined, 25–26
  durability, 83
  effectiveness/validity of, 90–91
  essential, 81–84
    Do Not Resuscitate (DNR) form,
      53, 88–89
    Financial Durable Power of
      Attorney, 25, 89–90
    HIPAA Authorization and
      Release, 69, 85–86
    Living Will, 25, 86–88
    Medical Durable Power of
      Attorney, 25, 84–85
  granting the right powers, 91
  hospital admission, forms to sub-
    mit, 187–88
  law firm, size of, 93
  lawyer versus online forms for, 82,
    91, 93
  original versus copies, 92
  recap, 94
  renewal/re-execution of, 84
  signing and witnessing, 91
  with and without, what happens,
    81–82
Power of Attorney
  agent/personal representative, 22,
    83
  definition/description, 83
  durability, 83
  medical, 25, 84–85
    accessibility of documentation,
      92

  access to medical records, 84–85,
    311n32
  agent/personal representative
    designation, 22, 62
  lack of, consequences, 82
  renewal/re-execution of, 84
  submission at hospital
    admission, 185
  versus Living Will, 88
  POA abbreviation/acronym, 83
  property (financial), 25, 89–90
    agent/personal representative
      designation, 22, 65
    annual re-execution, 84
    death of principle (loved one)
      ends power, 89–90
    documentation accessibility, 92
    lack of, consequences, 82
    proxies/agents named in, 22, 83
    renewal, need for, 84
    renewal/re-execution of, 84
    See also Power Documents
Pre-need contracts, 238, 239
Preston, Tom, 32, 262, 265, 317n97
Prognosis, 23, 143
  versus forecasting, 141, 145–46
  See also Forecasting
Proportionality, principle of, 264,
    317n99
Proxy, 26, 83

Q
Questions, 65–67
  asking the right people, 73
  asking your loved one, 68
  DNR conversation, 186–87, 193
  as documentation, 68–70
  end-of-chapter prompts, 75
  for hospital, DNR conversation,
    186–87
  hospitalization, front-end (fore-
    casting), 146–48
  if/else, 287
  for nursing staff, DNR conversa-
    tion, 191

Patient's Bill of Rights and, 72
question-asker role, 67–70, 74–75
question-asker role, building comfort with, 76–77
"what if?," 68–69, 75
See also end-of-chapter prompts

R
Racial issues, 169–70, 272–73, 317n104
Rationing, health care, 274–75, 316n95, 317nn106-7
Reading recommendations, 303–8
Records, medical. See **Chart; Medical records**
Records, personal representative's, 68–70
Reform, 273–74, 284–90
of end-of-life options, 256, 273–74
hospice/palliative care eligibility, 290
hospital administrative (recording of deaths), 285
of medical system, 246, 273–74, 284–90
patient-family autonomy, 290
patient-family resources, 285
ethical resources in hospital, 285
on-call ethical assistance, 285
patient-family treatment, 286–90
abandonment of treatment, inquiring why, 289–90
communication algorithms, 287–89
control over dying, 290
disclosure about resuscitation, 287
effective pain management, 286
forecasting, 286
ICU access, 24/7, 286
monitoring for symptoms of dying, 287
physician training and licensure, 284
end-of-life training, 284

palliative training, 284
See also Option to Die in PEACE
Refusing treatment, 111
leaving a hospital, procedure for, 174–75
Registered nurse (RN), 153–54, 167
Religiously based hospitals, 155, 312n40
Religious personnel
author's interviews with, 35–36
hospital chaplains, 139–40, 154–56, 285, 313n55
hospital mission directors, 106, 155, 312n40
Representation, effective, 55–76
See also Personal representative; Power Documents
Responsibility for problems, 292–93
Resuscitation, 52–53, 88, 187–96, 311n34
coding (Code/Full Code/Code Blue), 192
conclusion and recommendations, 210–12
definition/description, 189, 314n64
disclosure about, reform suggested, 287
DNR. See Do Not Resuscitate (DNR) conversation
effectiveness of, 196, 314–15n68
ethical gray zones, 196–211
future choices, 209–10, 315nn75-6
no-CPR directive, 89
practicalities and legalities of, 189–96
provider viewpoints and, 204–8
real life, messiness of, 193, 314n66
recap, 212
stopping, after it is started, 192–93
treatment goals and, 187–89, 205
unexpected circumstances, 197–201
See also Do Not Resuscitate (DNR) conversation
Rilke, Rainer Maria, 242, 247, 283, 316n86, 318n109

Roles
  caregiver, 71, 119
  dual/multiple, 59, 74
  question-asker, 65–67
Rounds (doctors'), hours of, 41, 147,
  162, 164, 165, 314n58

S

Schiavo, Terri, 150, 185, 1886, 255,
  314n62
Self-directed dying, 248–49
  See also Patient-directed dying
Self-restraint, diminished, 235
7 ten-thousandths, 263–64, 317n98
Shock, 37, 142–45
  absence of forecasting and, 139,
    142, 144–45
  definitions, 24
  extrinsic, 24, 143–45
    abrupt communication and, 143
    absence of communication and,
      103–4
    acute effects of, 143–44
    DNR snafus, 179–82, 196–201
    harm of, 144, 284, 293
    impact of accumulated, 175
    as improvised explosive device
      (IED), 175, 314n60
    poor communication and, 37
  intrinsic, 24, 142–43
  toll on family, 74
  unnecessary, 139, 143
  See also Forecasting
Snafus, DNR, 196–201, 289–90,
  315n70
  See also Do Not Resuscitate (DNR)
    conversation
Social worker, 153
Sonnet II:XIV **(Rilke),** 283, 318n109
Sonnets to Orpheus, The **(Rilke),** 242,
  247, 308, 316n86
Specialist liaison, 153
Spouse, access to medical records,
  69, 311n28
Stiff **(Roach),** 308

Stress, caregiver, 71, 268, 317n102
Suffering/bodily distress, 164,
  314n57
Suicide, 248, 262
  moot for the terminally-ill, 262
Surgery
  delays in, 164
  intubation and, 199–201, 205–8
  "operate or die" snafu, 198–201
  Power Documents and, 81
  recission of DNR order during, 194,
    199–201, 207
  who performs?/who is in OR?,
    168–69
Symbolic language, 235
"The system," 245
  as a moving target, 295–97
  changes in, 245–46
  patient-family as part of, 275
  reform of, 246, 273–74, 285–90
  understanding, 46–47
  See also Healthcare system

T

Taboo subjects, 243–44
Tape recorder, 69
Technician, nursing, 167
  firing, 171
Ten Tenors, 282, 318n108
Terminology/definitions, 19–27
Terri Schiavo case, 150, 185, 186,
  255, 314n62
Testing, delays in, 164
The Joint Commission. *See* **Joint**
  Commission, The
Theses of this book, 36–37
3 Secrets Hospitals Don't Want You to
  Know **(Meaney),** 32, 155, 304,
  318n111
Time
  active timing of hospitalized
    deaths, 256–58
  for body to respond, 164
  compressed time frame, 270
  in crucible, 263–64, 270, 317n98

delays in hospitals, 168
demands, for personal representa-
    tive, 70–71, 73
of doctor' rounds, 41, 147, 162,
    164, 165, 314n58
elasticity of experience, 245
Hospital Time, 148, 162, 164–66
self-directed dying and, 249
Time-based trial, 25, 204–5, 211, 289
To Die Well (Wanzer), 309
Training, physician, reforms
    suggested for, 284
Treatment, 105
abandonment of, questioning,
    289–90
discussions/conferences, 128–29,
    141
goals, resuscitation and, 187–89
hospice and, 252
need for family to oversee, 126
plan, 145
reforms suggested for, 286–90
refusing, 111
term use, 22
who provides?, 147, 167–70
See also Reform
Treatment group, 97
conflicts/impasses with, 150
defined, 22
end-of-life decisions and, 256–57,
    316n93
forecasting and, 145–46
language/conversing with, 69
number of clients/case load, 107
Power Documents and, 81–82
See also Hospital maze
Trusts (legal documents), 90

U
Unattended deaths, 236–37, 316n82
"Unsayable sum" of moments, 242,
    316n86
Un-word, 27, 309n10
Urgency to act, 53
Uustal, Diann B., 32, 141, 203

V
Variables, 51
Ventilating. *See* **Intubation**
Veterans, internment in VA
    cemetery, 238–39
Vital sign, pain as, 251, 285
Voice recorder, 69–70

W
Will (Last Will and Testament), 90
    relative cost of, 90, 312n36
    See also Living Will
Windrum, Bart. *See* **Author (Bart**
    Windrum)
"Wrong turn," dying unexpectedly
    due to, 249–50

Y
You: The Smart Patient **(Roizen, Oz,**
    and The Joint Commission), 306

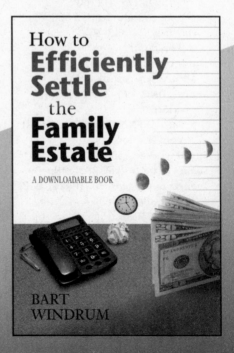